Y0-AAC-895

Population
Growth
& Health

Health and the Environment
Books in This Series

Population Growth & Health

Kim Etingoff

AlphaHouse Publishing
New York

Health and the Environment
Population Growth & Health

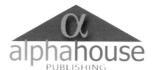

AlphaHouse Publishing
A Division of PEMG Publishing Group, Inc.
201 Harding Avenue
Vestal, New York 13850
www.alphahousepublishing.com

First Printing
9 8 7 6 5 4 3 2 1
ISBN: 978-1-934970-38-6
ISBN (set): 978-1-934970-34-8
    Library of Congress Control Number: 2008930665
Author: Etingoff, Kim

Cover design by Wendy Arakawa.
Interior design by MK Bassett-Harvey.

Printed in India by International Print-O-Pac Limited

 An ISO 9001 Company

Contents

Introduction

"The word *environment* does not mean something that surrounds us but an organism of all life within which we are fastened."
—Mose Richards, in
The Cousteau Almanac (1980)

Discussing the environment, we tend to speak as though it were a separate entity. "Protect the environment!" we demand, overlooking that *we* are an inseparable part of the environment. The air we breathe, the water we drink, the trash we discard, the sunlight to which we're exposed—all are different aspects of our environment. This series educates readers about humans' place in the environment and describes how intertwined our lives are with the natural world. Readers will also learn how certain human activities are degrading our environmental life-support systems, disrupting natural ecosystems and endangering human health in the process.

Among those at greatest risk for serious illness due to environmental pollution are children, the elderly, and those living in poverty, with children bearing the greatest share of the burden. According to the United Nations Environmental Program (UNEP), the quality of a child's environment is one of the key factors as to whether he or she will survive the first few years of life, particularly in developing countries. The World Health Organization (WHO) cites statistics showing that each year more than three million children under the age of five die due to environment-related diseases. Those claiming the highest toll include:

- Acute respiratory infections, 60% of which are related to environmental conditions.
- Diarrheal diseases, 80%-90% of which are a result of contaminated drinking water and poor sanitation.
- Malaria, the vast majority of cases resulting from lack of adequate mosquito control.

Such problems can only be solved through better environmental management programs. According to the WHO, preventing environmental disease could save the lives of as many as four million children each year. This series provides information on the health risks posed by environmental pollutants, describes ongoing prevention and management programs around the world, and offers useful advice to readers on how they can reduce their own risk of environmental disease.

Not only does this series describe how the quality of the environment affects us—it also explains how human activities affect the environment. Pollutants from automobile and factory emissions foul the air while wastewater from industrial discharges and inadequately treated sewage contaminate waterways. Improper disposal of hazardous materials and municipal solid waste can contaminate soils and groundwater, while careless use of chemical pesticides presents hazards to both humans and wildlife. Pollutants encountered in tobacco smoke, food, and water have been blamed for an increase in cancer rates and intestinal diseases. Humans create chemicals and wastes that foul the environment and these pollutants, in turn, can make humans sick. In addition, human population growth puts a steadily increasing strain on ecosystems, making environmental cleanup even more of a challenge.

Perhaps the greatest environmental threat of all is global warming. The predicted increase in violent weather, droughts, rising sea levels, spread of insect carriers of disease, crop failures, and resulting civil unrest will have a profoundly negative effect on people and the environment everywhere in the world.

We all need to learn how to make changes now to prevent irreparable damage to our atmosphere and our planet before it's too late. This series explores how the creation of new government policies and environmental laws is helping to bring about change and discusses how individuals can have a positive impact in their own homes and communities.

— Anne Nadakavukaren

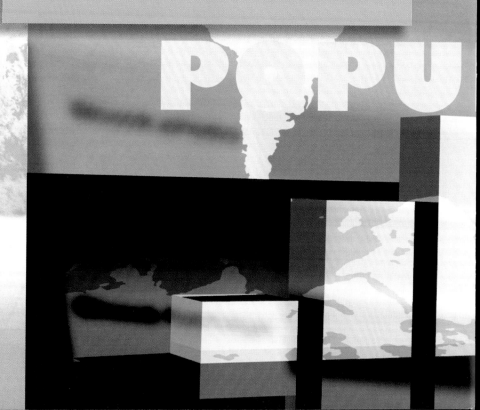

Here's what you need to know

- Population growth is the increase in the number of people in a given area that occurs when the birth rate is larger than the death rate.
- Population remained mostly steady on Earth until the eighteenth century and the Industrial Revolution, when the number of people grew exponentially.
- Today 6.7 billion people live on Earth.
- The rate of population growth is beginning to slow down; this is due mainly to the availability of contraception.
- Developing countries have the highest rates of population growth, for many reasons.
- No one knows exactly how fast the population of the planet will continue to grow, but most estimates say that the number of people will increase to about nine billion people before the population stabilizes.

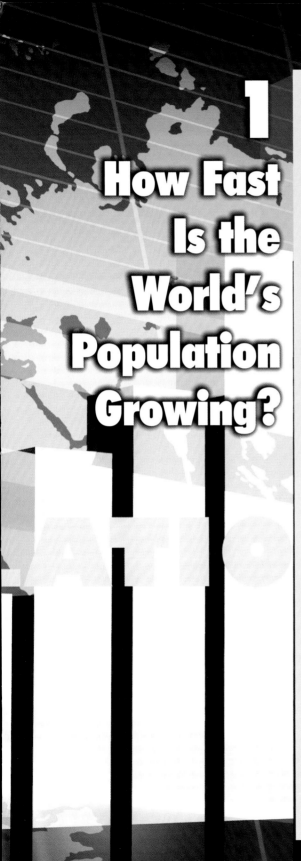

1

How Fast Is the World's Population Growing?

While it might seem like a grim list, our world faces many global problems such as natural disasters, climate change, and the HIV/AIDS epidemic. Behind these, however, lies a hidden issue: population growth. The sheer number of people on the planet makes such diverse crises as hurricanes and poverty worse every year. The more people there are, the greater the density of humans on earth, and the more resources that everyone must compete for. So, for example, in the event of a natural disaster, greater amounts of food and medical aid need to be shipped to victims in need. More people also means a struggle for land, drinkable water, oil, and other important resources that the world has a limited supply of.

The earth's population is now well over 6.5 billion people, and is still growing fast. However, there are signs that it is not growing as quickly as it has in the past, for a variety of reasons. But while growth rates might be slowing down over time, the total number of people will continue to rise for the next several decades, or even centuries, posing a serious dilemma for all of those additional people who must share space on the planet.

What Exactly Is Population Growth?

Essentially, the growth of any population, whether it is human or any other living creature, happens when its birth rate is greater than its death rate. Birth and death rates are usually defined as the number of either births or deaths per one thousand organisms in one year. When the balance between new members and dying members tips in favor of those being born, the population grows. On the other hand, if more members die than can be replaced by new members born into the population, it declines.

However, it's more complicated than that, and factors such as food supply, availability of land, and natural disasters affect the growth of a population. Outside influences can change both birth and death rates, which results in changes in growth. If, for example, the **fertility** of a population increases while its death rate is steady, growth will occur. This could happen if the food supply suddenly increases because of a stretch of good weather, or because of better child health care. If, however, the birth rate remains the same and **mortality** increases, the population will get smaller. A country dealing with HIV/AIDS or another widespread disease might experience something like this.

In terms of people, estimates of total world population are of interest, but growth is often broken down by country or region. It is important to distinguish populations by country or area. The population of Germany is made up of a different **demographic** than the population of Ghana, so they face different problems and require different solutions. Population growth in a specific area also sometimes includes migration, besides the number of births in that area. Many countries' numbers are increasing today because people from other parts of the world move to that area, not just because its citizens are having children. When those immigrants have their own children, the population then rises even further. Immigration

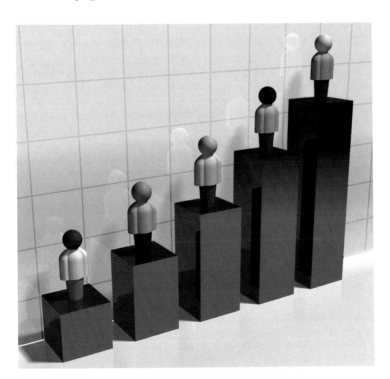

The World's population continues to rise with a projected increase to approximately nine billion people by the year 2050.

can be a country's only source of population growth, as in some European nations.

Population Through History

Even though the number of humans has been increasing at an enormous rate during recent history, this wasn't always the case. Two-hundred thousand years ago, our planet was the home to only a few thousand people. Even two thousand years ago, at the beginning of the Common Era, there were probably only about 300 million of us, which approximately equals the number of people living in the United States today. It has been estimated that during the 1000s, global population grew only by ten million, an astonishingly small rate considering how fast the human population is growing today. In fact, up until 1500, people were added to the population at less than 0.1 percent per year. This lack of growth was due to the high incidence of death because of disease, accidents, and lack of food.

All of this changed in the eighteenth century. Population grew in the wake of better knowledge of agricultural

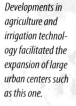

Developments in agriculture and irrigation technology facilitated the expansion of large urban centers such as this one.

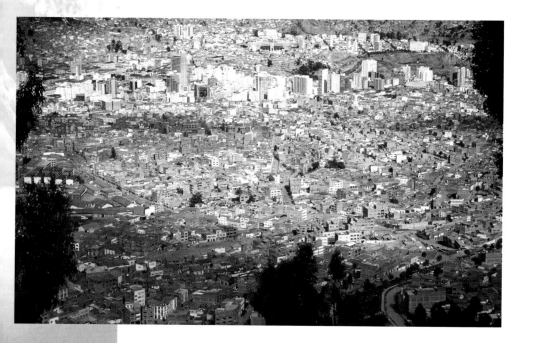

methods and technology that increased how many crops we could grow. The first signs of the enormous growth that would occur during modern times arrived with the Industrial Revolution of the late 1700s. Improvements in agriculture that boosted food supplies, better public sanitation, and advances in medical science drastically lowered death rates, setting the stage for rapid population growth. During the next two hundred years, growth increased to 0.5 percent per year, yet this was still insignificant compared with what was to come. Starting in the mid-twentieth century, **developing** countries began to have greater access to more productive methods of agriculture and new forms of medicine. Combined with the increasing **standard of living** in **developed** countries, population growth rates shot up to over two percent per year in the 1960s.

Two percent may not seem very big, but in terms of human population, it equals tens of millions of people each year. It took us thousands of years to reach the one billion mark, but only 123 years to get to two billion. Even more astounding, it was only thirty-three more years until we numbered three billion; we then doubled that and reached 6 billion people in 1999. Yet another half billion people were added in only nine years, so that the population of the world in 2008 was greater than 6.5 billion and is continuing to grow.

Population Today

After the boom leading up to the 1960s, population growth slowed down. During the 2000s, it has reached about 1.2 percent per year, which translates to about 76 million more people every year. Fertility rates are still higher than the replacement rate at this pace of growth. In order to remain stable and neither grow nor shrink, the human population must have a total fertility rate of 2.1. In other words, every pair of people must have about two children to replace them. The number is slightly higher than two, because some people will die before they can have children. Countries that fall below this rate will decline in number while those that have higher birth rates will increase. Population growth has slowed in part because several countries have fallen below this replacement rate. As of 2008, women in as many as seventy-three countries had fewer than an average of 2.1 children each. But more important, the growing number of people on the earth can be partly explained by the fact that many more countries' replacement rates are still well over 2.1.

There are almost 6.7 billion people on the planet (slightly less than half are female), but of course that number won't stay the same for long. Right now, the most populous country is China, at 1.3 billion, but India is a close second and may soon surpass China, with almost 1.2 billion. The United States comes in third, but has a far smaller population than either China or India, with about 300 million people. Fourth and fifth are Indonesia and Brazil, with approximately 237 million and 192 million, respectively.

Part of the reason for the slowing of the growth rate is **contraception**, also known as birth control. Women, as well as men, all over the world now have available and effective ways of avoiding unwanted pregnancies, making families smaller. Increasing availability of things such as condoms, birth control pills, and sexual health education have been allowing couples to avoid unwanted pregnancies. Globally, the average number of children per woman was 2.6 in the years between 2000 and 2005. This was down from an average of 4.5 children per woman thirty years earlier. Increasing use of contraception would likely decrease fertility rates even more, slowing down population growth.

Another trend in the world population is aging. For probably the first time in history, the number of older people looks to be surpassing the number of children: in 2007, 11 percent of the population was over 60. It has been predicted that the older population will be larger than the population of children beginning in 2047, because the number of older people has been growing at a faster rate than world growth in population as a whole. Today, the average age of everyone on Earth is 28, but because of aging, the average is estimated to be 38 by 2050. This trend brings a lot of changes with it, adding to the problems associated with population growth in general. There are economic consequences, such as increased costs of health care; social changes and changes in the makeup of families; and political changes, all because of aging populations.

Many of the world's people, young and old, live in cities. In fact, a majority of people now calls an urban area home. As of 2007, more than half of the population lived in urban areas, and that figure is likely to remain true into the future. Many people are being driven out of rural areas because of food shortages, war, or other reasons, and are looking for better opportunities in cities. As a result, a large part of the world's population increase is happening in urban areas.

The Roman Catholic Church's opposition to artificial birth control methods, such as oral contraceptives, has influenced population policies of some majority Catholic countries such as the Philippines, where in 2000 birth control pills were banned from city-funded clinics in the capital of Manila.

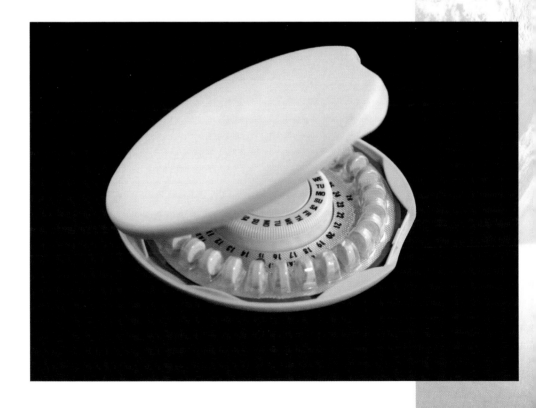

Not All Population Growth Is Equal

Average figures of population growth can be deceiving. There are actually vast differences in growth rates between different areas of the world. As with the distinctions between cities and rural areas, countries have varying growth rates. Nations are usually classified as either developed or developing. In the past, they might have been called first- and third-world countries, but both sets of terms refer to the amount of **industrialization** in each country. The part of the world referred to as developing, or as having less industry, is much larger. Over five billion people live in more than one hundred developing countries, while about one-sixth of the total population lives in about sixty developed nations.

Today's population growth is fueled in large part by developing countries, which include the two largest countries in the world, China and India. Birth rates are very high in developing countries, where the fertility rate is up to or more than five children per woman. These areas traditionally have less access to and education about contraceptive methods, although this is beginning to change. In Chad, only 3 percent of women use contraception, much less than the world average of 63 percent. However, the difference in contraceptive use between developed and developing countries is not always that great. Many developing regions have high rates of contraceptive use—above 60 percent—but places like sub-Saharan Africa, Micronesia, and Polynesia still have levels below 30 percent. Developing countries also have larger urban populations than their developed counterparts; 90 percent of urban growth is in these countries.

The populations of developed countries, on the other hand, have stabilized over the past few decades. All

Ask the Doctor

Q: My brother says that we don't have to worry about overpopulation, because there is still plenty of open space left and the six billion humans there are can all fit onto the Isle of Wight. Somehow this seems a bit silly, but I can't put a finger on why.

You're definitely right in thinking that it all sounds a bit silly. Although you can pack a lot of humans into a telephone booth, it doesn't mean that they can actually live in there. Even though our actual population can be greatly compressed, our carrying capacity can't, and that is remarkably close to being too much for the planet.

together, the people living in these countries number about 1.2 billion, less than 20 percent of the total population. Small growth is still occurring though, at around 0.2 percent a year. Compare this with 2.36 percent a year, the growth rate of the continent of Africa, and you can see the different problems developed and developing areas of the world face. Many developed counties are even experiencing a decrease in population, if immigration isn't taken into account. It is estimated that by 2050, several countries, including Germany, Japan, and Italy will actually have smaller populations that they do today.

All over the world, but especially in developed countries, the sizes of households are dropping. In 1950, developed countries had an average of 3.6 people per house, but in 1990, there were 2.7. In these areas, people are generally marrying later, waiting to have children, choosing to have fewer children, or are getting divorced, all of which encourage smaller household sizes. Use of and knowledge about contraception has also been high for several years, contrasting with the relatively recent increase in the use of contraception in developing countries, so developed countries have a head start in stabilizing their populations.

Did You Know?

Today, the country with the highest rate of population growth is Liberia. The Cook Islands have the lowest rate of population growth; their populations are actually shrinking!

According to the CIA World Factbook, Liberia's estimated population growth rate for 2008 is 3.6%.

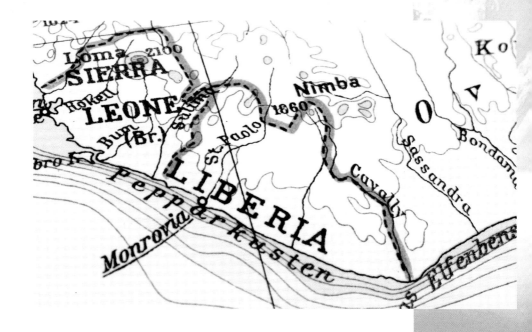

Developed countries also have older populations. The aging of the world population is due mainly to the growing number of older people in developed countries, as opposed to aging in developing countries. Advances in health care have extended people's lives at the same time that fertility rates have dropped, so the number of older people has caught up with and surpassed the number of children, beginning in 1998. In more industrialized nations, more than one-fifth of the total population is over 60. In the near future, developing countries are expected to follow the same trend, and there will eventually be twice as many older people in the world as there are children.

What the Future Holds

Scientists are unsure about what the future holds for us in terms of population. It's likely that human population growth will continue throughout this century, but whether there is an end in sight to that growth is impossible to predict with any certainty.

Most people agree that population growth is at least slowing. The UN Population Fund estimates that there will be approximately 9.2 billion people in 2050, an increase of 2.5 billion from today's numbers. Developing countries will make up an estimated 7.9 billion of that. While that may seem like an enormous jump in numbers in just four decades, if the population were to grow as fast as it is currently, there would be 10.6 billion people in developing regions alone by 2050.

Urban areas will probably increase by two billion people over the next twenty-five years, so that by 2030, two-thirds of all humans will be living in cities. Meanwhile the rural population will decline by 20 million, as more and more people choose to or are forced to move out of their rural homes and into the city.

Along with the uncertainty about how fast we will continue to grow, there are various guesses as to how many people the earth can hold based on space and availability of resources such as food and water. Many people have come up with estimates of the Earth's **carrying capacity**, the maximum number of people that the globe can support. Some researchers claim that we have already reached and gone beyond the number of people that can live comfortably together and with a healthy population, while others have come up with a higher estimate of carrying capacity. In addition, the Earth could support a lot more people with a lower standard of living, so while 33 billion people could live minimally on the planet according to the Food and Agriculture Organization, only a few billion could be supported with better lives.

Most estimates suggest that the population will probably increase to around nine billion people before it stabilizes, although that is an uncertain guess. But even if those estimates prove true, with nine billion people on the planet, we will continue to face huge problems such as providing universal health care, water and food shortages, and pollution.

India is home to some of the world's most populated cities, such as Mumbai and Delhi. These vast metropolitan hubs put overwhelming strain on environmental and socioeconomic resources; among them are health care delivery systems that are unable to keep apace with the rapidly expanding cities.

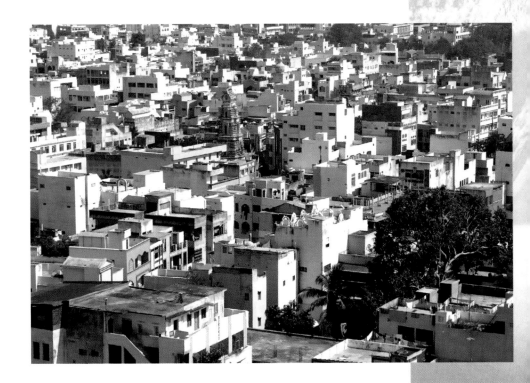

STRAIGHT FROM THE SOURCE

The UN Population Fund releases a yearly report titled The State of World Population. In 2007, the report focused on the increasing urbanization of the population.

In 2008, the world reaches an invisible but momentous milestone: For the first time in history, more than half its human population, 3.3 billion people, will be living in urban areas. By 2030, this is expected to swell to almost 5 billion. Many of the new urbanites will be poor. Their future, the future of cities in developing countries, the future of humanity itself, all depend very much on decisions made now in preparation for this growth.

While the world's urban population grew very rapidly (from 220 million to 2.8 billion) over the 20th century, the next few decades will see an unprecedented scale of urban growth in the developing world. This will be particularly notable in Africa and Asia where the urban population will double between 2000 and 2030: That is, the accumulated urban growth of these two regions during the whole span of history will be duplicated in a single generation. By 2030, the towns and cities of the developing world will make up 81 percent of urban humanity.

Urbanization—the increase in the urban share of total population—is inevitable, but it can also be positive. The current concentration of poverty, slum growth and social disruption in cities does paint a threatening picture: Yet no country in the industrial age has ever achieved significant economic growth without urbanization. Cities concentrate poverty, but they also represent the best hope of escaping it.

What Do You Think?

- How can cities help people escape from poverty?

- Why might the concentration of poverty in cities be a bad thing?

- Why do you think people are moving to the cities, resulting in this huge amount of urban growth?

Find Out More

To learn more about these topics, check out these Web sites:

World Population Awareness: www.population-awareness.net

UN: www.un.org

US Census Bureau: www.census.gov

World Bank: www.worldbank.org

Population Resource Bureau: www.prb.org

Here's what you need to know

• The more people there are, the more doctors and other health care workers are needed. This can be a problem especially in less-developed countries, where the number of medical professionals is far less than the number of people who need their services.

Words to Understand

The **health care industry** is all the people, resources, and technology that are used to care for the population.

Maternal health care is the medical attention that mothers receive during and immediately following pregnancy.

A person's **life expectancy** is how long they are expected to live. This is based on a variety of factors, including genetics, job, nutrition, and health.

The word **prenatal** means before birth; for example, prenatal care is attention that is given to a baby before it is born.

A **communicable disease** is one that is easily spread or transmitted from person to person.

An **epidemic** is when a disease quickly spreads throughout a large area and affects many people at the same time.

• Older people require more and different health care than the general population. This means that as a population ages, more medical workers are needed to fill these specific roles.

• Family planning is essential to reduce population growth and to ensure that mothers receive the appropriate prenatal care.

• Urbanization can lead to the development of city slums, where health care is generally poorer than it is in the majority of the city.

• Medical systems that are already spread dangerously thin because of population growth can become even more ineffectual when HIV/AIDS is brought into the picture; people affected by this disease need much more care than many systems can give them.

2
Population Growth and Health Care Delivery

The number of people on Earth is clearly growing at an impressive and alarming rate, but how exactly does this impact those of us who are individually part of that increasing population? One effect that everyone may eventually feel is the way that population growth shapes the health care people receive around the world. Additional people put a strain on the **health care industry**, stretching our medical resources thin. Doctors, nurses, hospitals, drug companies, and other professionals and groups involved in delivering health care will have to serve greater numbers of people as time goes on. Already, millions of people worldwide don't have access to the necessary health care, and die from diseases that could have been cured with the right treatment. As everyone competes for medicines and hospital care, some people, mainly the poorest, will not receive the care they need.

Health Care for the Masses

For countries dedicated to providing health care for their citizens, population growth equals trouble. More health care workers are needed to serve the millions of people added each year, whether it is in emergency medical care, dentistry, reproductive health care, or family medicine. In many cases, the rate at which the number of medical workers grows lags far behind population growth. Nurses, especially, are in short supply, but are a crucial part of caring for the millions of people flooding doctors' offices and hospitals. If there aren't enough medical workers, those people will go without proper health care, and wounds, infections, and diseases will remain untreated.

This aspect of population growth is certainly not limited to developing countries. Studies done in Canada, for example, showed that the number of health professionals fell by 1.7 percent in the decade between 1988 and 1997. Although there were more specialist health care workers such as chiropractors, the number of doctors and nurses per person fell, leaving some Canadians with more limited medical care.

A growing population also puts a strain on the budgets of countries with health care programs. Public health care programs—those that are run by governments rather than private companies—require government investment to work properly. The more people who rely on these programs, the greater the financial strain on the government, and the quality of health services may suffer as a result. Governments have many other worries besides health care and must decide what programs to back with money. A developing country in Latin America might face the tough decision of whether to spend limited money on industrial development that could improve thousands of lives, or to spend it on **maternal healthcare**, which would also help thousands of mothers and children.

The Problems of Aging

Besides the simple fact that there will be more sick people to attend to and provide care for, population growth and

The high cost of health care is a worldwide concern. Even in wealthy industrialized countries, such as the United States, nearly 47 million people are un-insured, forcing many to make difficult choices between investing in basic life necessities or seeking preventative medical care.

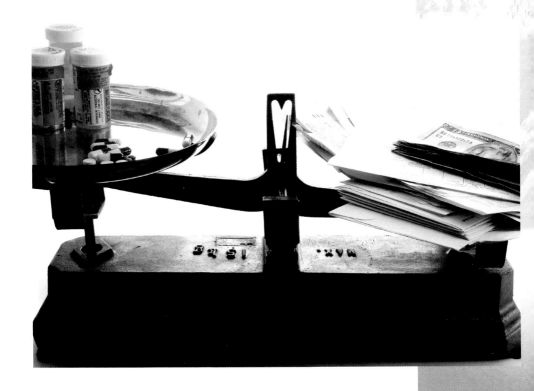

Did You Know?

Only 3% of married women in Chad are using contraceptives.

The rise in global life expectancy has put increased pressure on health care systems worldwide as elderly populations require greater medical attention or care.

changes in population also bring a different set of problems. The aging of the world's population has especially powerful effects on the health care industry, since older people generally need more medical attention. As the population gets older, particularly in developed regions, aging persons will expect and require medicines and medical procedures to help them into their old age. Diseases and conditions that affect mainly older people, such as many types of cancer and heart disease, are serious problems that require a great deal of time, resources, and effort to treat.

Also, more people are living longer, adding to the burden being placed on global health care systems. **Life expectancy** is much higher than it has ever been, since medical care has in fact improved over the past several decades. Today, the average person can expect to live to about 65, but in some countries, life expectancy has risen above 80 years old. Certainly extending the age of the

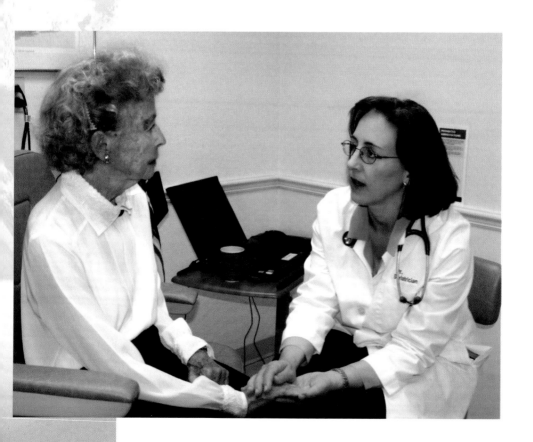

world's population is seen as a positive thing; the problem lies in how fast global life expectancy has increased, which has left many countries unable to deal with their aging citizens. There aren't yet enough health care workers, facilities such as nursing homes, or ways to support older people financially, and this dilemma will need to be addressed as the aging trend continues.

Family Planning and Reproductive Health

One of the roots of population growth is fertility. While some women are having fewer children, those in developing countries are continuing to have an average of as many as seven children each. (Niger has the highest fertility rate in the world, at 7.1.) Many people have tried to address this issue, tackling education and action surrounding family planning. Family planning, which includes contraception, refers to the conscious decisions made to limit the number of children in a family. Government programs, international health agencies such as the World Health Organization (WHO), and nonprofit organizations are all seeking to reduce the number of children per woman in hopes of slowing or stopping population growth.

According to the UN Population Fund (UNFPA), at least 200 million women are lacking effective ways to plan families and use contraception. Without access to contraception, even women who want to have fewer children are unable to. Family planning might be unavailable because of the lack of government programs, the absence of medical clinics, or the high cost of care.

One area of the world where family planning is at the forefront of humanitarian efforts is Africa. As a region, Africa contributes substantially to the world's population growth: it currently has a growth rate of 2.5 percent per year, while other developing areas of the world, such as Latin America, have lower growth rates. In many developing areas such as Africa, modernization has changed the way that people plan families. Traditionally, African cultures offered women many ways of choosing to space their children, such as periodic abstinence, but modernization has changed the mind-set of many of Africa's women and men. Now, the problem is introducing contraception and providing education on family planning.

Reproductive health goes along hand-in-hand with family planning. It refers to health issues surrounding pregnancy, such as **pre-natal** care. Millions of mothers give birth to children every year, but some face greater danger than others. UNFPA estimates that difficulties related to reproductive health are the number-one cause of death and illness in women who are of childbearing age. Although women in both developed and developing countries die during childbirth, the number is significantly higher in developing ones, where reproductive health care isn't as available. Women who are poor and malnourished are more likely to have complications during pregnancy, often give birth to unhealthy babies, and frequently become disabled or die because of the birth.

Hospitals and clinics that must already deal with too many sick or injured people do not have the time or resources to take adequate care of the many women who need good health care while pregnant. Family planning would therefore also ease the burden of health care facilities, leaving them free to give others better medical attention and to make sure that the births that do happen are safe.

Ask the Doctor

Q: Our family farm barely has enough acreage to support my husband, my two children, and myself and that is with both my husband and myself working all day. Although it has been two years since we have had a child, I am deathly afraid of the hardship my family could endure if I do get pregnant again, as there will be another mouth to feed and I will be unable to work the farm for several months. However, my husband refuses to wear a condom. What can I do?

You are right to see birth control as a potential solution to this problem, although the fact that your husband refuses to do his part is a problem. However, there are other options available, such as oral contraceptives, spermicidal creams, or female condoms. There are aid organizations that can help get them to you. Go to your nearest community medical clinic for help finding the right resources.

Urbanization

The urbanization of developing countries is usually seen as a positive step forward, since nations that are more urban have historically been more prosperous. However, the rapid movement of people from rural areas to cities can have harmful health costs. Cities don't always have the capacity to house and feed more people, so slums develop. Slums are very poor areas of a city that generally have bad sanitation, insufficient housing, and a very dense population. They are frequently unhealthy places to live, as many thousands of densely packed people spread **communicable** diseases, drink unsanitary water, and are unable get the right amount or kind of food to eat.

Health care in slums is also not always sufficient to take care of slum populations. Cities are hard-pressed to provide so many people with health care, since they are

The growth of impoverished urban slums is one consequence of cities that are overburdened by the rapid pace of internal migration from rural areas to urban centers. The risks of spreading communicable diseases are elevated in slums due to inadequate sanitation and insufficient access to health care.

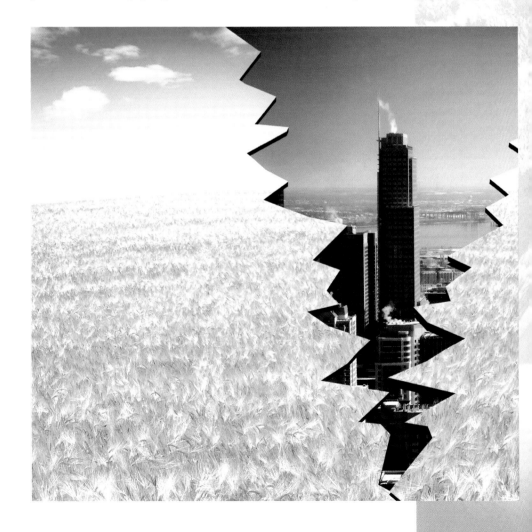

both poor and in danger of many health-related issues. The high density of people living in slums makes it difficult to pay enough medical attention to the thousands packed into small areas, even if some health care is available.

HIV/AIDS

According to the 2007 UN World Population Policy report, most countries belonging to the UN consider HIV/AIDS as their main population concern. Ninety-three percent of developing countries reported that the **epidemic** was a major concern, and so did an almost equally high percentage of developed nations. Some estimates suggest that there have been over 25 million deaths related to the disease, and millions more carry HIV, making it a truly global problem that affects economic development, family structure, food production, and health.

Because there are so many people in the world today, it is difficult to give everyone with HIV/AIDS the attention they need. Developing countries especially are overwhelmed with the thousands or millions of citizens who need health care to treat the disease. The hardest hit area of the world is sub-Saharan Africa, a region already struggling with economic development along with a growing population. In some African countries, at least a fifth of the population is living with HIV/AIDS. In places such as sub-Saharan Africa, where so many people are overwhelming a health care system that isn't equipped to deal with a disease of this scale, people aren't getting treatment. For a number of reasons, including high prices for medicine and the enormous number of people in need of health care, less than a third of all people in developing countries received a form of care called antiretroviral treatment in 2006. HIV/AIDS is an urgent problem on its own, but combined with population growth, it equals devastation.

STRAIGHT FROM THE SOURCE

The World Health Organization has a six-point agenda that guides the organization in addressing health issues around the world. It's third stated goal is strengthening health systems, in order to provide better health care to people in every country. It reads:

For health improvement to operate as a poverty-reduction strategy, health services must reach poor and underserved populations. Health systems in many parts of the world are unable to do so, making the strengthening of health systems a high priority for WHO. Areas being addressed include the provision of adequate numbers of appropriately trained staff, sufficient financing, suitable systems for collecting vital statistics, and access to appropriate technology including essential drugs.

What Do You Think?

- How might adequate health care affect population growth?

- What might prevent some countries from developing health care systems on their own?

Find Out More

To learn more about this topic, check out this Web site:

World Health Organization: www.who.org

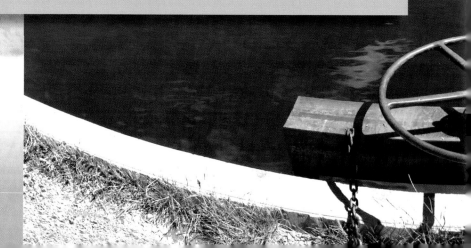

Here's what you need to know

- Although 70 percent of the Earth is covered by water, most of it is in the oceans, where we cannot use it to drink or to feed crops.

- In the past few decades, the demand for water has increased dramatically.

- Many less-developed countries are having problems providing enough water for all their citizens. However, developed countries are facing problems as well, especially in areas that are naturally dry and hot.

- The increase in agriculture has meant that a greater amount of the available water is being used to grow the crops that are necessary for human survival.

- Population growth has led to an increase in pollution, especially along waterways. This can mean that people's only source of water becomes dirty and can cause severe health problems.

- Everyone needs fresh water, so countries have tried various ways of bringing water to people; these methods include taking water from aquifers and treating the wastewater so it becomes suitable for human consumption.

- When water is scarce, it becomes a valuable commodity that people are willing to fight over to obtain.

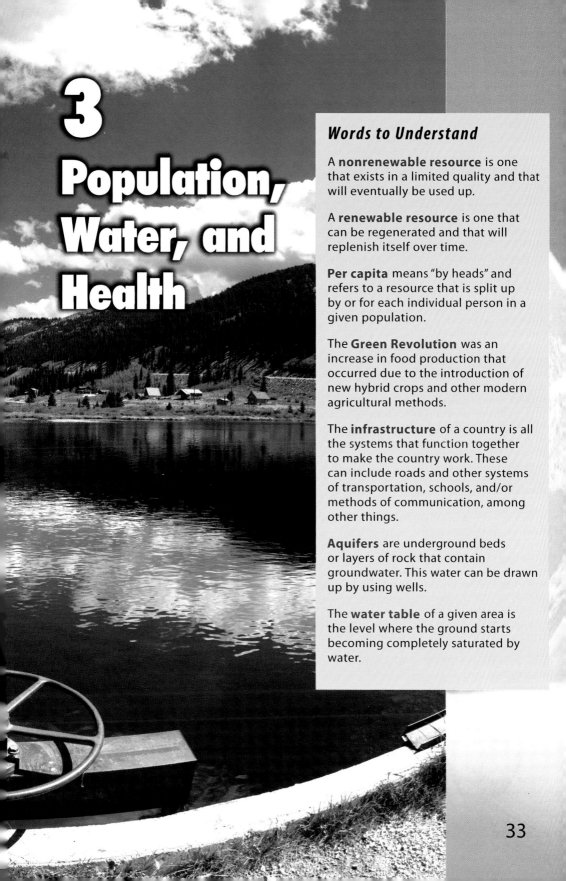

3 Population, Water, and Health

Words to Understand

A **nonrenewable resource** is one that exists in a limited quality and that will eventually be used up.

A **renewable resource** is one that can be regenerated and that will replenish itself over time.

Per capita means "by heads" and refers to a resource that is split up by or for each individual person in a given population.

The **Green Revolution** was an increase in food production that occurred due to the introduction of new hybrid crops and other modern agricultural methods.

The **infrastructure** of a country is all the systems that function together to make the country work. These can include roads and other systems of transportation, schools, and/or methods of communication, among other things.

Aquifers are underground beds or layers of rock that contain groundwater. This water can be drawn up by using wells.

The **water table** of a given area is the level where the ground starts becoming completely saturated by water.

While the number of people may be growing, our natural resources are not. Unfortunately, the planet doesn't expand with the population, and we must work with the limited resources that the Earth already provides us with. **Nonrenewable resources** such as fossil fuels and minerals are not increasing to match the addition of millions of additional people every year who rely on them. Nor are there more **renewable resources**, such as trees, solar radiation, and wind. The availability of fresh water, a renewable resource, is one of the most pressing concerns for humans. Every person needs a certain amount of water to survive, and trying to stretch the available water supply to cover the needs of billions of people is an ongoing challenge.

We might turn on our faucets or drink from water bottles every day without thinking twice, but all over the world water scarcities are a reality. Water isn't just used for drinking or for personal use. It also plays a big part in agriculture, since animals and crops must also consume water—much more than humans, actually. It has been estimated that over 60 percent of water used goes toward

The world's burgeoning population continues to force policymakers and scientists alike to search for innovative ways to harness renewable energy and decrease societies' dependence on nonrenewable, and environmentally unfriendly resources, such as oil.

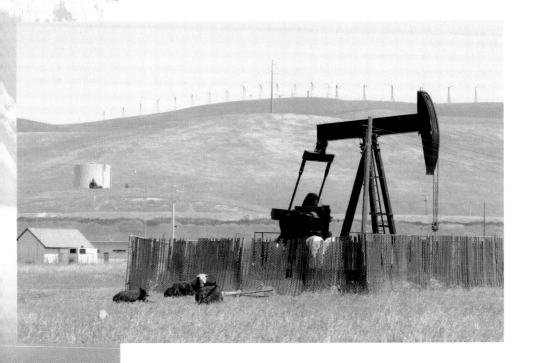

the watering of crops, but that number can reach as high as 90 percent in some countries with large agricultural production, such as China. Water also adds to the quality of life; luxuries such as warm showers, bottled water, and hot tubs are comforts that some people would find hard to live without.

About 70 percent of the globe is covered with water, but most of it is contained in the oceans. Despite its abundance, this water is mostly undrinkable because it is so salty. Only 3 percent of all water is considered freshwater, but over half of that is trapped in the form of ice in glaciers and at the polar ice caps, or is located deep within the Earth's crust. That leaves about 1.5 percent of the world's vast water resources available for human consumption. Regardless of this small percentage, that 1.5 percent still equals trillions of tons of water that is recycled through the ground, atmosphere, and bodies of water every year. That's plenty of water to sustain a modest population of people, but it's not enough as we reach past the six billion mark.

Increased Demand

Over the past few decades, the demand for water has increased dramatically, mirroring and even outstripping the growth of the population. Since 1970, an additional two billion people have reduced the **per capita** availability of water by one-third. In other words, there is two-thirds the amount of water today for each person, on average, than there was forty years ago. The demand for water has not, in fact, increased proportionately to population: it has grown even faster. While population tripled during the 1900s, the same time span saw a sixfold increase in the demand for water.

This can be explained by increasing needs not only for drinking water, but also for agriculture and industry, as well as leisure and recreation. Part of the reason for this rise was the **Green Revolution** of the mid-twentieth century, which led to a large jump in food production, increasing the amount of water needed for agriculture and the operation of agricultural machinery. The world as a whole also eats more meat, which has added to the demand for water. Raising one kg of beef uses 13,000 liters of water, while the same weight in potatoes needs only 100 liters. Nor is there a much better outlook for the future: the UN has estimated that by 2050, approximately 4 billion people will be experiencing water scarcity, a little under half of the total number of people that are expected to be living then.

Lack of water is sometimes defined in terms of water stress and water scarcity. If a country has less than 1700 cubic meters per person, it is probably water stressed. Below that level, there are likely either temporary or permanent shortages of water every year. Water scarcity is even more extreme—less than 1000 cubic meters per person—and can have serious consequences for health, industry, and economic development. Individually, people need at least 100 liters of water a day, plus up to twenty times more for industry and agriculture. Anything less than this cuts into water used for drinking, bathing, growing food, or industry.

Since the amount of water on Earth isn't growing, population growth is putting a lot of stress on what we do have available. In the five years between 1990 and 1995, 125 million more people were added to water-scarce countries, putting even more of a strain on the rest of the populations of those areas. As of 2002, the World Health Organization estimated that at least 1.1 billion people already had limited access to freshwater for drinking, and the number grows every year as more people are added to the population.

The Inequality of the Water Supply

Lack of water is a global crisis brought in part by population growth, but not all parts of the world face the same shortages. Water is distributed unevenly across the continents, and some countries simply have more access to water than others because of the way our planet formed and because of natural rainfall levels. Rivers, lakes, and springs provide many nations with water, but some have little or no way of getting freshwater. In general, countries around the equator and some northern regions have enough water, sometimes even an excess of it. Other places, especially Africa, are naturally very dry, and can't provide enough water for those who live in the region. No access to rivers or lakes, or minimal amounts of rainfall, makes water hard to come by for drinking and cooking, much less agriculture or industry.

Region by region and country by country, population usually does not match water supply. Asia, for example, has over 60 percent of the world's people, but only about 35 percent of the world's water from rivers. By contrast, South America has a very small percentage of the population, but 26 percent of the water supplied by rivers, including one of the world's longest rivers, the Amazon. In many instances, the countries that face the severest water shortages are among the world's poorest and least developed.

Water pipes like this one deliver drinkable water to communities who might not otherwise have access to clean water sources. Many people in developing countries are without access to safe and clean drinking water, which increases their risk of contracting waterborne diseases.

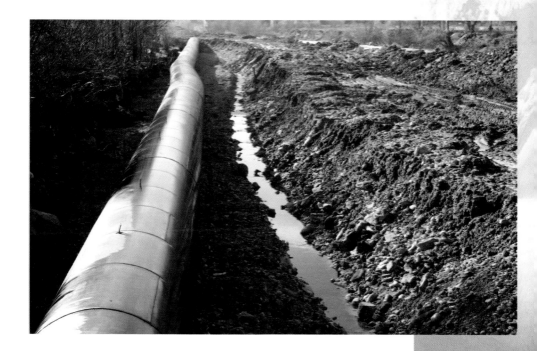

However, developed countries are by no means free from water scarcity problems. Regions of the United States, especially in the southern and the naturally dry western portions, are facing water stress, as more people are born in or move into cities and the suburbs surrounding them. Atlanta, Georgia, for example has seen a huge growth in population and is also at the mercy of droughts. Georgia certainly can't grow its own water, so it has had to fight other surrounding states for control of some rivers to provide Georgians with more freshwater.

Irrigation

Dry areas of the world are hit hard for two reasons. Many dry countries, such as Egypt, have large growing populations and must use a large amount of water just for private consumption. Second, dry areas do not have much rainfall to water crops, so agriculture uses up enormous quantities of water that could otherwise be used by individuals in homes. The necessity for food and water is the same in these dry nations as in wetter ones, but they don't have the

Irrigation is an unsustainable water management technique.

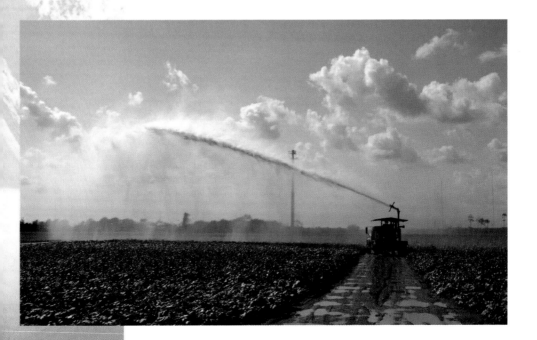

same access to freshwater resources and must find ways around this problem.

Irrigation all over the world uses up a large percentage of freshwater resources, and in most countries, watering crops uses up much more water than that used for drinking. Asia, with about two-thirds of the world's irrigated cropland, uses about 85 percent of all its water for the irrigation of its crops. Rivers are diverted for the sake of irrigation, usually by dams, affecting their courses and sometimes drying them up. Similarly, lakes and inland seas such as the Aral Sea in Central Asia are even emptied by massive irrigation projects.

Nor is irrigation a very effective method for producing food. Usually, irrigation methods are very inefficient and end up using much more water than is really needed to grow crops. It is estimated that less than half of the water used actually reaches the roots of the crop being watered, since much of it is lost to evaporation and poor design. Irrigation can also cause salt to accumulate in fields, which reduces how much crops produce. Irrigation is also one reason that agriculture is so harmful to the environment and to human health. In India, tens of thousands of square kilometers of land have been left vacant because overuse and improper irrigation design has made it uninhabitable and not suitable for growing food. Right now, irrigation accounts for over sixty percent of freshwater use, so every bit that is wasted limits how much is left for drinking water, industry, or other agricultural activities.

Lack of freshwater impacts health on many levels. Besides the need for water used directly for drinking, people also desperately need enough water to produce food. Dehydration and malnutrition threaten the segments of the world population who don't have access to either or both, putting them in danger of disease or death.

Some people fear that water will eventually be commodified, meaning that people will have to pay money for the use of water. A larger population puts a huge strain on the amount of water we have, so as it becomes more valuable, it will become a part of the global marketplace.

If this happens, the poorest people will have very limited access to water, since it will be another added necessary cost in their lives. Once water is commodified, health issues related to the lack of water will likely turn into an even greater threat.

Pollution of Water

Besides the fact that more people means less water for each, the growth in population has lead to the contamination of a number of freshwater resources. In many cases, pollution from the sewage produced by billions of people contaminates water with bacteria and viruses, making it unsafe to drink. It is estimated that as much as ninety percent of the world's sewage is dumped into bodies of water without first being treated. Diseases such as cholera can then be spread through this infected water. According to the World Health Organization, 3900 children die every day from diseases spread by the contamination of water. Water ecosystems around the world are also destroyed by polluted water. The harmful pollutants can eventually move up the food chain from bacteria to fish to human, indirectly influencing the food supply of people all over the world.

More people also equals more stuff. The demand for more goods means that someone has to make those goods, which in turn can lead to pollution of freshwater. Factories often dump waste into oceans, lakes, and rivers, since that is sometimes the easiest way to get rid of unwanted byproducts. Like sewage, a huge percentage of industrial waste is dumped directly into sources of freshwater. Again, the pollution introduced in places where fish or other aquatic food is caught can potentially sicken humans.

The urbanization of the population also affects water quality around the world. A lot of people in one area produces large amounts of waste that can contaminate the limited sources of water available to people who live in cities. Also, the rapid population growth in urban areas doesn't mean that **infrastructure** in those cities has caught up. The means of getting freshwater to people in cities often just don't exist, so city-dwellers have to drink from contaminated sources of water, getting sick in the process.

Dealing with Water Shortages

The enormous number of people needing water has lead to drastic actions. People simply can't live without freshwater, so many countries have tapped into varying ways of getting the most out of what their resources hold. One of the most common methods of getting more water is withdrawing it from rivers as they flow by. So many people use the water diverted from rivers such as the Nile in Egypt, the Yellow River in China, and the Colorado in the United States that they don't even reach the sea.

Although there are other options, they pose their own problems. Some countries or areas turn to the treatment of wastewater to reuse as safe drinking water or as industrial-grade water. This decision costs a lot of money, though, and might not be realistic for all countries. Another option is underground reserves of water that can be drilled into and brought to the surface. Along with water withdrawal from rivers, using water from **aquifers** has grown by up

THE GREEN REVOLUTION

The Green Revolution of the mid-twentieth century brought both benefits and more problems to the world. Beginning in the 1940s in Mexico, the scientists and policymakers involved in the Green Revolution promoted the use of new hybrid crops, new agricultural machinery, irrigation, and pesticides. These things increased the amount of food grown to feed the world, combating hunger in places that traditionally had less access to food. However, the Green Revolution also meant things such as more pollution and over-irrigation. The benefits of the Revolution were also not distributed equally among everyone, leaving behind the extremely poor. Today, hunger and malnutrition are still such problems that it is clear we need to use other methods to tackle feeding the world's population.

to 3 percent a year since 1940, reflecting the growth of the population. Unfortunately, this isn't a problem-free answer to water scarcity. Pumping water from the ground lowers the **water table**, which impacts the land above, making it unstable. In the short term, withdrawing water from the ground gives people access to freshwater, but in the long run, possibly lowering the water table can be dangerous for the local environment, as well as for the people living in the area.

Unintended Consequences: Conflicts Over Water

Added to the stress caused by population growth are the conflicts that are brought on because of the need for water. Since freshwater is a resource that is needed for actual survival, countries, states, and individuals often have to fight for it. All over the world, but particularly in water-starved Africa and the Middle East, people are entering into conflicts over water. Tension builds between nations looking to have control over a particular source of water, whether it is the start of a river, a lake, or a supply of groundwater. Over 260 rivers alone are shared by at least two countries, and all hold potential for provoking conflicts as the population continues to grow and water resources are stretched to the breaking point. This tension sometimes worsens relations between regions that may already be in conflict. Israel and Jordan, Turkey and Iraq, Sudan and Egypt, and India and Bangladesh are only a few examples.

Ask the Doctor

Q: Our farm has for generations used the same well for our source of water, because the land that we work is rather dry and we need the water for irrigating our crops. But these past few years, there's been less and less water coming out, and other wells that we've dug haven't produced anything more. Now, we don't have enough water to bring in our regular crop, and we're losing money. What's going on?

The well that your farm was using probably was drawing water from an underground aquifer. However, that water in the aquifer is almost all used up, and its replacement will likely take thousands of years. The other wells that you dug have the same problem because the original well had probably drawn up all the water over a wide area, like someone drinking up soup from a bowl with a straw.

STRAIGHT FROM THE SOURCE

The WHO recognizes the importance of having enough clean water for everyone on Earth to use for drinking, bathing, cooking, and recreation. Among the many facts it lists on its Web site are:

Poor water quality can increase the risk of diarrhoeal diseases including cholera, typhoid fever, salmonellosis, gastrointestinal bacteria, and dysentery. Water scarcity may also lead to diseases such as trachoma and typhus. Trachoma, for example, is strongly related to a lack of water for regular face washing.

Water scarcity encourages people to store water in their homes. This can increase the risk of household water contamination and provide breeding grounds for mosquitoes—which are vectors for dengue, dengue haemorrhagic fever, and malaria and other diseases.

What Do You Think?

• Why might people not have access to clean water?

• Why do you think water scarcity makes people hoard water in their homes?

Find Out More

To learn more about these topics, check out this Web site:

World Water Council

www.worldwatercouncil.org

Here's what you need to know

- Starvation occurs when people don't get enough to eat; eventually their body will break down all the stored fat and tissue in an attempt to get enough energy to survive.
- Malnutrition is when a person's food does not contain the right combination of nutrients; this is the most common health problem in the world today.
- A third of all the people in the world are affected to some extent by malnutrition; however, these people are mostly concentrated in less-developed countries, like Africa and parts of Asia.
- How much food, as well as what kinds of food, we eat has changed in the past few decades. Today, people are demanding more meat, fruit, and vegetables, and fewer staples such as cereal and rice.
- Because of a growing population, the food needs of a growing population have been met by increasing yields per acre, largely through increased use of fertilizers, pesticides, and better crop varieties.
- We are in the midst of a global food crisis today; the rising price of food will eventually force many people into poverty.

Words to Understand

Emaciation is the condition of abnormal thinness that is caused by malnutrition or starvation.

Anemia is a blood condition where the cells cannot carry enough oxygen to the rest of the body. While there are many causes of anemia, including genetics, it is often caused by not consuming enough iron.

Immune systems are all the parts of human bodies that work together to prevent diseases from getting a foothold in the body.

Imports are things that are traded in a country from other countries; they are brought in for the purpose of being bought and sold.

Something that is **stunted** is slowed or stopped in growth before it has fully developed.

A **staple** is a basic item of food. Foods such as flour and rice are often considered staples.

An action that is **unsustainable** is not capable of being maintained or supported for an indefinite period of time.

4
Population, Food, and Health

Although people can't survive without water, they also need to eat food to stay alive. However, unlike water, humans can control and increase how much food they have access to, choosing to grow more to feed a growing population. Of course, these sorts of choices have consequences, and the impact that the need for more food has on the world is significant.

As the population grows, there is naturally an increase in the demand for food, since there are more mouths to feed. The UN estimates that by 2030, food demand will have doubled since 2008, at least 20 percent of which is due to population growth. But food is a complicated resource. In addition to the relation between increasing population and demand for food, there are many other factors involved in calculating and predicting how much food the world's population will need. Age, distribution of population, culture, and expectations about quality of life are all important determinants of how much food a country or region needs.

Nevertheless, there is a certain amount of food that a person needs to eat to live. Without the nutrients that foods contain, there is no way to survive. We need things such as protein, vitamins, and minerals to grow and stay healthy, fight diseases, and remain strong. But population growth puts pressure on the world food supply. For a number of reasons, not everyone gets enough to eat, or all of the nutrients needed for a healthy diet.

Starvation and Malnutrition

There are many health issues related to the availability of food. Some people simply don't get enough to eat and face what is called starvation. If the body doesn't receive enough energy and nutrients, it eventually breaks down stored fat and tissue, leading to **emaciation**. Many health problems result, such as reduction in muscle mass, diarrhea, **anemia**, low body temperature, and shrinking organs. People who consistently do not receive enough food will likely die. Starvation is most common in very poor regions of the world, especially in developing areas.

No less serious than starvation is malnutrition. People whose diets are lacking in the right combination of nutrients, or who do not get the right amount of food to eat, are said to be malnourished. Where the global food supply is concerned, malnutrition is the main health-related issue facing the population today. It is a condition that strikes when a person doesn't get the right nutrients, or the right amount of food, and occurs commonly not only in developing countries, but in developed ones as well.

There are actually several different kinds of malnutrition. Undernutrition, also called protein-energy malnutrition, is the result of an inadequate intake of calories for

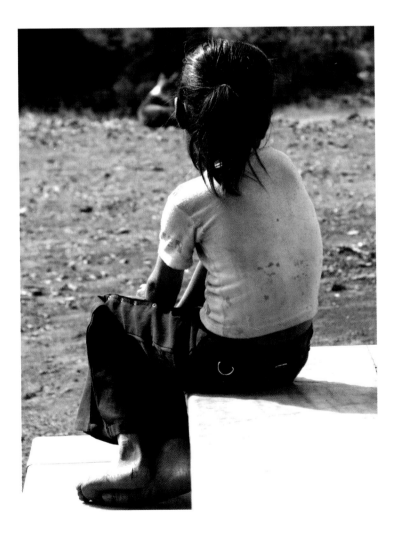

According to the FAO, roughly six million children die from malnutrition every year.

energy and protein; overnutrition, often in the form of obesity, is its opposite, resulting from too many calories. Other specific types of malnutrition include secondary malnutrition, when a person's body is unable to use the food they eat because of a disease or illness, especially diarrhea.

The effects of malnutrition can be devastating. Death is a very real consequence of severe malnutrition because people's bodies are unable to function without enough nutrients. Mothers die during childbirth because of malnutrition, and many millions of people die from diseases that attack their weakened **immune systems**. Other problems include birth defects in children born to mothers with malnutrition, decreased mental capacity, and underdevelopment.

Distribution of Malnutrition

Like population growth itself, malnutrition is unevenly distributed across the globe. According to the World Health Organization, in 2000, one-third of all people were affected by malnutrition. By far, most of these people were concentrated in developing countries, where access to water and good sanitation, as well as food, was the least likely. At the turn of the millennium, about 70 percent of children, the age group most affected by undernutrition, lived in Asia, while most of the rest lived in Africa. Developing countries are also the sites of the most rapid population growth; the two trends are in fact closely related. The causes of hunger mirror those of lack of freshwater.

Other factors, however, are also important in explaining why developing regions have a higher rate of malnutrition. Hunger and malnutrition are quite often a product of poverty, which is itself often related to large concentrations of people in small areas. Developing countries with growing populations are among the world's poorest nations, and don't have the infrastructure to educate people about nutrition or to provide them with the options to choose a variety of food that would prevent malnutrition. In developed nations, poorer people usually have less access to nutritious food, and are at higher risk for malnutrition. Climate works against populations, too: parts of Africa, for example, are naturally arid and don't offer the same abundance of food that other areas of the world take for granted. As of 2008, the U.S. Food and Agriculture Organization listed 36 countries as having a food security crisis. Twenty-one of those countries were in sub-Saharan Africa, a region that relies heavily on food **imports** because it is difficult to grow crops such as wheat and rice.

Malnutrition also strikes people of different ages differently. Children are most vulnerable to the effects of malnutrition: over 50 percent of the deaths of children under five are because of this condition. Children especially need good nutrition to help them grow and stay healthy while growing. Without the proper types and amounts of nutrients, children easily fall prey to diseases and illnesses. In developing areas of the world, 10 percent of children are classified as having the most severe form of malnutrition. Thirty percent are **stunted**, one of the effects that malnutrition can have on growing children. Other groups that are also at an increased risk of the consequences of malnutrition include pregnant women, breast-feeding women, and the elderly.

Changing Food Needs

As the population becomes more urbanized and experiences rapid change, the kind and amount of food that people eat is changing. How much meat we eat in particular is growing, but people are on average also consuming more fruit and vegetables. Globally, people ate thirteen more kilograms of meat in 1998 than forty-five years earlier in 1963. On the other hand, **staple** crops such as cereals and rice are not as large a part of people's diets as they once were.

The amount of food that we eat has also increased. In the 1960s, the average person ate about 2300 calories per day. Near the end of the millennium, we ate almost 2800 calories a day. Total number of calories wasn't the only thing to increase either: intake of individual nutrients such as protein has also jumped during the twentieth and twenty-first centuries.

There are also factors working against the increasing demand for food. The aging of the global population plays a role in how much food we eat, and could act as a trend that counteracts rising demand. As humans age, we naturally need less food to go about our daily lives. Worldwide, the population is aging, which could have a significant impact on how much food the world actually needs. Another factor involved in a decrease in food demand is the nature of people's lifestyles. People who are physically active for most of the day, such as farmers, need more food to keep them going. Today, more people are working at jobs and leading lives that don't include a large amount of physical activity.

Land Crunch

Competition between a growing population and the need for food production is leading to a shortage of land. The density of the population—how tightly packed people are into a specific area of land—directly affects how much land is available for growing crops. In places such as eastern China, where the population density is quickly rising and industry is squeezing out agricultural land, growing food has become a real problem. Between 1988 and 1995 alone China lost almost one million hectares of cropland to construction.

Added to the rapid loss of land is the fact that the land that is already being used for the production of food is being exhausted. Over the years, farming the same land over and over has depleted the quality of the world's soil, making it less productive. This type of farming is **unsustainable**, reducing the amount of land that humans can use to grow crucial food. By 1990, it was estimated that 38 percent of all cropland was degraded, in addition to 21 percent of pasture and 18 percent of forests. In fact, one estimate claimed that the productivity of croplands is 12.7 percent less than it would otherwise be because of human agricultural activities.

Livestock's Role

Animals kept for the purposes of eating or for providing products such as milk are a major contributor to the world hunger problem. Livestock need a lot of food and water to grow, taking away grains that would otherwise go directly to feed people. Because the demand for meat is growing along with the population, millions of kilograms of corn and soybeans are used to fatten up livestock for meat or dairy production. In order to make a profit, many farmers are growing crops to feed to livestock rather than people.

The Recent Food Crisis

Recently, food prices have begun to soar, plunging the world into a global food crisis. A number of factors have contributed to rising food prices, especially the cost of staple crops such as corn and rice. Lower agricultural production because of unsustainable farming practices is one major reason: as the population grows, demand for food is rising, but crop output is not, driving prices up. There have been no major increases in crop yield in the past few years either. In the past, new technologies or techniques were developed in agriculture that helped farmers produce more, but that has not happened in recent years. Changes in weather patterns also prevented agricultural output from keeping up with population growth. Our energy demands are yet another big factor in rising food prices. The price of oil has steadily risen, making the transport of food and water much more expensive, which then translates into higher food prices.

For millions of people around the world already struggling to buy enough food to stay full and healthy, rising food prices are definitely not a welcome problem. Without

Real People

Glenn used to be a teacher of sustainable agriculture several years ago. He often took his students on extended trips to South Africa, where they learned about agriculture in the field. On one trip, he was invited to the village of a man who lived in the area; he agreed to go and spent the night in the man's home. While there, he met the daughter of his host, a little girl named Ida, who was obviously very sick from malnourishment. She had just returned from the nearest hospital, but her family was still very worried about her.

The next day, Glenn returned to the village he was staying in with his students. Soon after, he was told that Ida had died in her home. Her village was plunged into grief, and her father mourned for his daughter's loss. Although the people who lived in the area were probably not strangers to the deaths of children because of malnutrition or disease, it didn't mean that this child's death was any easier.

About a year after Glenn's return to the United States, he was contacted by Ida's father. He and his wife had a new baby that they wanted to name after Glenn. Declining the offer, Glenn agreed instead to name the baby himself, and chose the name Joy, hoping it would bring luck to the couple. Unfortunately, a few months later, he received the news that Joy, too, had died of malnutrition.

OBESITY AND MALNUTRITION

You may not think of obesity as a form of malnutrition, but obesity and overweight result from getting the wrong kind of nutrients. Instead of not getting enough nutrients, people who are obese get too many of them, or eat the wrong kinds of food. Obesity is a problem in both developed and developing nations, and affects all social and economic classes. It is quickly becoming one of our most serious nutritional issues, since it leads to illnesses such as heart disease, diabetes, stroke, and cancer.

rising incomes to match the costs of food, many people will have to cut some or most of their food choices out of their diet, leading to more malnutrition and more starvation. In some parts of the world, such as Kenya, people spend 80 percent of their income on food. If that food increases in cost, they are not able to afford as much. Corn, the major food in Kenya, has doubled in price, leaving many people able to buy only half of what they could previously buy.

The World Bank estimates that food prices will stay high until at least 2015. That's plenty of time to force more people into poverty because they can't afford to buy food. The Bank estimates that if the price of rice in Indonesia were to rise by just 10 percent, two million more people would become poor. It's the same story all around the world; the poorest people who are currently managing to live on what money they make will be the first to feel the effects of rising food prices.

STRAIGHT FROM THE SOURCE

The World Bank has created a plan to address the growing food crisis. Some of its main points are included below, but there are many more.

The World Bank Group's New Deal on Global Food Policy has been endorsed by 150 countries. The New Deal embraces short, medium and long-term responses: including safety nets such as school feeding, food for work, and conditional cash transfers; increased agricultural production; a better understanding of the impact of biofuels; and action on the trade front to reduce distorting subsidies and trade barriers. The Bank is taking action by:

Creating a $1.2 billion rapid financing facility to speed assistance to the neediest countries.

Boosting overall agricultural lending to $6 billion over the next year.

Launching risk management tools and crop insurance to protect poor countries and small-holders.

Nearly doubling agricultural lending to Africa from $450 million to $800 million; and to Latin America from $250 million to $400 million.

Supporting over $1 billion in new projects in agriculture and rural development in South Asia.

Doubling lending for social protection, nutrition and food security, and social risk mitigation to $800 over the next year.

What Do You Think?

• Why might understanding how biofuels work help address the food crisis?

• What are some of the connections between food security and trade barriers?

Find Out More

To learn more about these topics, check out these Web sites:

GAIN
www.gainhealth.org

Food and Agriculture Organization of the UN
www.fao.org

Here's what you need to know

- There are several types of air pollution; the most common are air, water, soil, light, and thermal pollution.
- There are various sources of these types of pollution, although most pollution is produced by human activity.
- Water pollution can lead to waterborne diseases such as cholera, and air pollution can lead to respiratory illnesses.
- Lead, which causes brain and nerve damage, is found in leaded gasoline, old paint, and some soil.
- Pollution in developed countries is usually nonbiodegradable, or chemical, but pollution in developing countries is usually biodegradable, or biological.
- Individual as well as governmental support is key in reducing the amount of pollution that the world generates.

Words to Understand

Thermal is of or relating to heat.

Something that is **fatal** causes death.

Sediment is made up of loose particles of sand, silt, or clay suspended in water.

Pathogens are microorganisms that cause infection or disease.

Particulates are tiny particles of liquid or solid suspended in the air.

Neurological refers to the nervous system, which includes the brain, spine, and nerves.

Eutrophication is the process in which a body of water receives too many nutrients, which leads to an overgrowth of plant life, which strips the water of oxygen.

GDP is the Gross Domestic Product, which is the total value of all of the goods and services within an individual country.

5
Population and Pollution

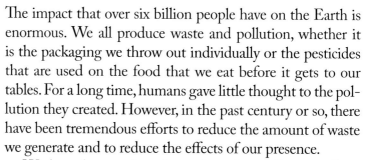

The impact that over six billion people have on the Earth is enormous. We all produce waste and pollution, whether it is the packaging we throw out individually or the pesticides that are used on the food that we eat before it gets to our tables. For a long time, humans gave little thought to the pollution they created. However, in the past century or so, there have been tremendous efforts to reduce the amount of waste we generate and to reduce the effects of our presence.

We have known for a long time that pollution affects both the environment we live in and our own health. Adding chemicals and other wastes to the environment leads to all sorts of health problems. They range from relatively minor ones such as coughing and headaches, to major medical concerns such as cancer, birth defects, or respiratory illness. Now, with ever-larger numbers of people being added to the globe, the impact of pollution is even more extreme, both in the amount of pollution that is produced, and the number of people pollution affects.

Pollution's Sources

The first attempts at pollution control were in response to water contaminated by human waste, and the smoke in small houses created by cooking and heating fires. People realized that waterborne diseases such as cholera and respiratory problems were caused by human activity, which provided an important incentive to change that activity. Sanitation measures have since been put into place in some parts of the world, as well as ventilation in small spaces, but many people are still in danger of both types of pollution.

Pollution usually refers to the contamination of the environment, mainly with manmade materials. It can be broken down into specific types of pollution, such as air, water, soil, light, and **thermal**. The first three of these are especially tied to health hazards, since people interact with the Earth's land, waters, and air continuously. Pollution is a difficult thing to avoid. People produce pollution individually—when they drive a car—and by purchasing or using things whose creation involved pollution—eating a tomato grown with pesticides. Humans always naturally produce waste, which must go somewhere after it leaves the body. If the waste enters a body of water for example, it has the potential to make others who drink the contaminated water sick. We also produce garbage, with some societies producing more than others. Garbage is particularly a problem in industrial developed areas, where people consume many products that have excess packaging, and where throwing away a product that is lightly used is normal. Garbage is also a huge problem in developing countries where people are now using plastic bags, tin cans, and other disposable packaging just as much as developed countries, but where local governments haven't yet begun to provide comprehensive waste collection and disposal services. Other human activities also create pollution, including the creation and use of energy, transportation, and agriculture.

Population growth is frequently the culprit of increased pollution. The more people there are using up resources, the more waste is generated. There are other factors as well, though. New technology as well as people's consumption habits are also responsible for creating more waste. If everyone on Earth expects to buy two TVs rather than one, it will have the same effect on pollution as if the population

There have been reported cases of wealthy industrialized nations illegally dumping vast amounts of hazardous electronic waste in developing countries to avoid the high costs of waste disposal within their own borders. In 2006, Cote D'Ivoire called for financial assistance from the United Nations Environment Programme to clean up contaminated sites caused by a ship that came from Europe and dumped waste there.

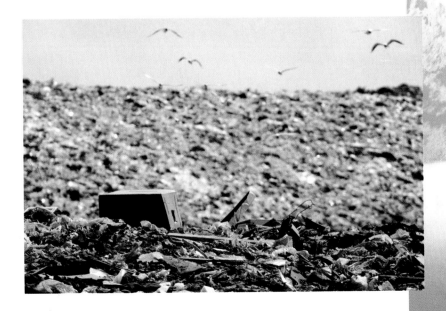

had doubled but only bought one TV. In the United Kingdom, people produce more than five hundred million tons of waste every year. That's equivalent to over eight tons of waste per person! In fact, studies have shown that population growth led to about a quarter of increased greenhouse gas emissions, while consumption led to the other three-quarters. Population growth was found as the main force behind increased methane emissions from agriculture. Although population growth may just be one of many factors involved in pollution, it is a very significant one.

Polluted Water

Water pollution is perhaps the most health-threatening type of contamination. Diseases such as dysentery, cholera, typhoid, and hepatitis, which are all potentially **fatal**, are waterborne illnesses. Infected water is the cause of two million deaths every year, as waterborne diseases travel through rivers, streams, and lakes where people get their drinking water. Children are very vulnerable; up to ten million children are infected with these types of diseases every year.

Contamination of water is a common problem throughout the world, both in developed and developing countries. Protection of water resources often falls by the wayside as other issues are tackled. In developed countries especially, water is usually purified after being drawn from the source, so that although people can get fresh drinking water, the bodies of water it comes from are still polluted. Meanwhile, in developing countries, the laws and/or technology to keep water from getting contaminated do not exist.

Agriculture is the main source of water pollution. Fertilizers used to increase crop yields, animal manure, and pesticides to keep insects off crops run off into rivers and lakes, affecting everyone who uses that water. Farming puts too many nutrients, **sediment**, and **pathogens** into the water supply, making it toxic for both aquatic life and humans. Even ten years ago, pollution from agriculture had contaminated almost 300,000 kilometers of water-ways in the United States alone.

Industry is another major player in water pollution, adding to the hundreds of chemicals that are estimated to be in rivers around the world. As with farms, factories also sometimes dump their waste directly into bodies of water, without regard for the environment or people's health. Acid rain, created by the release of sulfur dioxide and nitrogen from industry and cars, contaminates fresh water as well as land. As acid is added to the environment, toxic metals such as lead and mercury can be produced, which are dangerous chemicals for humans to ingest either directly or through poisoned fish and other food.

Air Pollution

Everyone is affected by air pollution. Unlike with water, we can't filter the air to get rid of contamination. Contamination of the atmosphere is caused mainly by industry, which releases pollutant gases and **particulates** into the air. Transportation is another huge source, as millions of people travel every day in cars, and cases of food and goods are shipped around the world on trucks, planes, and trains. The American Association for the Advancement of Science estimates that over half of the world's urban population is exposed to dangerous smog. Burning coal and exhaust from vehicles create what is known as smog—clouds of fog and gas that form on windless days, mainly in cities.

Smog, and other less visible air pollution, causes many respiratory illnesses and deaths every year. In China, 50,000 people die annually because of air pollution in just the eleven biggest cities. In addition, 400,000 people come down with chronic bronchitis every year. Other respiratory conditions, such as asthma, are triggered by air pollution. Air pollution has also been a problem for many decades, as the 4000 smog-related deaths in London in 1952 prove. Today, it is estimated that air pollution is connected to up to 50 percent of cases of chronic respiratory

Did You Know?

When Mount Saint Helens in Washington State erupted in 1980, ash from the eruption was found in the atmosphere all over the world within two weeks.

illnesses. Cities are taking drastic measures because of smog. Some cities, such as Mexico City, frequently end up closing down factories and moving cars and people inside when smog becomes too dangerous.

Smog and air pollution isn't just a problem where the contaminants are released. Winds move air pollution from its source to places many miles away, crossing state lines and the borders of countries. This leaves some areas dealing with health-damaging pollution that comes from a completely external source. Living out in the countryside isn't an escape from air pollution, either, since winds easily move smog from cities to rural areas outside of them.

Yet another source of air pollution is the burning of waste. Households around the world burn their waste to get rid of it instead of throwing it away, or burn wood to clear brush. However, this just changes potential pollution of land into air pollution. Burning waste releases chemicals called dioxins into the air, which can cause respiratory problems and cancer if they build up to high levels. You might be familiar with burn bans where you live: there are now widespread laws limiting how must waste can be

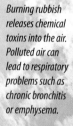

Burning rubbish releases chemical toxins into the air. Polluted air can lead to respiratory problems such as chronic bronchitis or emphysema.

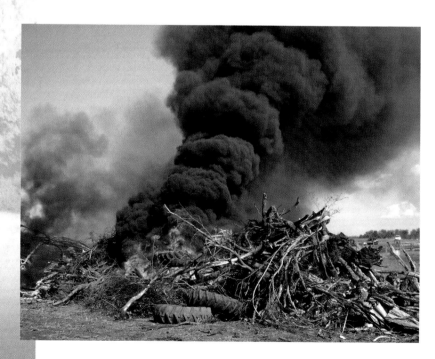

burned, especially if there is no wind to carry away the chemicals from the site of burning.

Lead Pollution

One of the most toxic substances to humans is lead, a metal that was used in consumer goods for many years until it was found to cause irreversible **neurological** damage. In children, who are the age group most often affected by lead exposure, lead causes brain damage, trouble learning, and stunted growth. Adults exposed to lead can have reproductive problems, muscle pain, and nerve disorders. Lead comes from several sources, such as exhaust from cars using leaded gasoline, old paint, and soil.

Countries such as the United States have banned lead from all products, but other nations don't yet have laws limiting its use. In large cities where people use gas with lead, many are poisoned with lead. In Africa's biggest cities, lead levels are up to ten times higher than in European cities, and as the populations of those cities grow, even more people will be susceptible to the health effects of lead.

Developed vs. Developing

There are different problems with pollution in different parts of the world, because of the presence or lack of industry, governmental regulations, and lifestyles. In studies done of historical pollution levels, it has been found that as countries begin to industrialize, their pollution levels go up. However, as they continue to industrialize and incomes rise, pollution levels often decrease, because people have the desire and money to pay for pollution regulations.

Many developed countries have put these regulations in place with positive results. Water, soil, and air quality are improving in developed regions of the world, as the levels of pollutants such as lead, sewage, and sulfur dioxide decrease. The stabilizing population levels in developed countries also have an impact on pollution. Since these nations aren't being overwhelmed with hundreds of millions of new people every year, they can figure out how to deal with the pollution produced by the population size they currently have. And if fewer people are being added to the population, contaminants introduced into the environment also decrease.

However, the news isn't all good for the developed regions of the world; they certainly still have their share of problems. Water pollution remains a big problem for Europe. In 1998, three-quarters of Poland's rivers were too polluted to use even for industry, which doesn't require the same standard of sanitation as water used for drinking. Groundwater too is being polluted with chemicals from agriculture and industry, a serious health hazard for those who use tainted aquifers. Europe's lakes, as well as North America's, are also experiencing **eutrophication** because of agriculture fertilizers containing nitrogen.

Developing countries face an even bigger problem. Even though not all developing nations face the same degree of pollution as developed ones because they have less industry, rapid population growth and lack of technology and infrastructure put billions of people at risk of health problems due to pollution. Usually developing regions have many issues to deal with, and the government may not always place cleaning up pollution, a big job in the best of cases, at the top of their list.

People who live in developing countries usually do not have the same access to sanitation as those in developed nations do. As a result, raw sewage and garbage is dumped straight into rivers and lakes without any treatment, spreading disease. In places such as Thailand, rivers have thirty to one hundred times the amount of bacteria and viruses than is deemed healthy by its government.

Pollution is also a different problem in developing countries because it actually involves different materials.

Ask the Doctor

Q I live along the shores of a lake where my family, my friends, and I fish for a living. Just a year ago, some men came out from the city and built a large factory on the shore, where we now send the fish we catch to be put into cans and sold in the city. However, there's one problem. The number of fish that we're catching has been decreasing, and some of what we do catch has these strange open sores. What's going on?

Unfortunately, the cannery is likely polluting the lake and killing the fish, as well as causing the survivors to have problems. Although your options are likely limited, find a different line of work and avoid eating any more fish from the lake if possible.

Studies suggest that pollution in places with lower incomes produces waste that is mainly biodegradable, such as food waste. In developed areas of the world, on the other hand, although some pollution is biodegradable, a much larger percentage is not. Instead, it is made up of manmade, mass-produced chemicals from agriculture, industry, and households that stick around for a long time. Neither type of pollution is necessarily any less dangerous than the other: biodegradable pollution can carry pathogens, such as the contamination in water systems. Nonbiodegradable pollution introduces foreign chemicals into the human body, and can lead to dangers such as lead or mercury poisoning.

The fastest-growing and fastest-industrializing countries are hit hardest with pollution problems. Nations such as India and China have populations of over a billion, but also are quickly becoming more industrial. There, governments and citizens have to deal with the effects of having more people every day producing waste, in addition to the increasing amounts of waste produced by growing industry and industrial agriculture. In India, all fourteen of its major rivers are polluted. In Pakistan's largest city, the sewage treatment plants cannot deal with the number of people recently added to its population. Most sewage leaks out into the ground and contaminates drinking water surrounding the plant.

Future of Pollution

Pollution is a particularly visible problem. We can see the effects that releasing chemicals into rivers or into the air has. Resources become dirty, animals and plants die, and people get sick. There is no ignoring incidents such as the dumping of over a billion tons of industrial waste into the Liao River in China in 1986, when every organism living in the river within 100 kilometers of the dump site died. And as the world becomes increasingly industrial, pollution is likely to increase. Rising incomes generally result in greater generation of waste. A study done of countries belonging to the OECD showed that a 40 percent increase in **GDP** was mirrored by a 40 percent growth in

Did You Know?

It was estimated that in 2007, 10 billion gallons of raw sewage were dumped into Lake Erie in the northeastern United States.

waste production. Many countries' GDPs are rising, and as an unfortunate side effect, their production of waste and pollution will also.

Fighting against this trend is an opposite one: technology and awareness. Although new technology can add to pollution, it can also reduce it. In the interest of saving money, as well as for environmental protection, companies have begun reducing packaging, so that consumers throw out less waste. In countries that have been industrialized for a long time, it has been found that there is less pollution per unit produced. Unfortunately, this hopeful sign is offset by the countries that are newly industrializing, and that do not have the experience or the money to limit their emissions. It is also offset by population growth. For example, in the United States, cars now emit less pollution per mile driven than in the past, but because there are so many people driving cars long distances, the United States continues to produce more and more air pollution from vehicles. Any gains we make in reducing how much pollution we create will automatically be overwhelmed by how many people there are on Earth producing waste.

Individual awareness of the problems of pollution also helps prevent pollution and its harmful effects on health. People have realized the dangers that contamination poses to health and the environment, and are taking active steps to fight it. Governments also play a role in creating legislation that prevents pollution and sets guidelines for sanitation and acceptable levels of contaminants in the water, soil, and air.

THERMAL POLLUTION

Thermal pollution usually refers to the damage done to water by a source of heat. These sources are often factories that spill excess industrial heat into lakes, streams, or rivers, although increasing the amount of sunlight that reaches water by cutting down trees or other vegetation can also cause thermal pollution. This type of contamination affects the oxygen content of water, changing the ecosystems that live off of stable oxygen levels, and killing many organisms.

STRAIGHT FROM THE SOURCE

As part of its work, the WHO is addressing indoor air pollution, which is especially a problem in developing countries where people cook in unventilated homes. Indoor air pollution is just as much of a concern as outdoor air pollution, particularly for children.

More than three billion people worldwide continue to depend on solid fuels, including biomass fuels (wood, dung, agricultural residues) and coal, for their energy needs.

Cooking and heating with solid fuels on open fires or traditional stoves results in high levels of indoor air pollution. Indoor smoke contains a range of health-damaging pollutants, such as small particles and carbon monoxide, and particulate pollution levels may be 20 times higher than accepted guideline values.

According to The World Health Report 2002, indoor air pollution is responsible for 2.7% of the global burden of disease.

What Do You Think?

• What are some other causes of indoor air pollution?

• Why is carbon monoxide so dangerous, especially in enclosed areas such as houses?

Find Out More

To learn more about this topic, check out this Web site:

www.pollutionissues.com

Here's what you need to know

- The United Nations is working on the issue of population growth by attempting to reduce poverty, provide safe reproductive services, and reduce HIV/AIDS in countries that need its aid.
- Some developing countries, such as China and Kenya, have official population policies that help to keep population growth in check.
- The UN, the World Health Organization, and other international organizations work to educate people all around the world about population growth and health.
- Politics, natural disasters, and a general lack of understanding are all obstacles the world faces in the fight against population growth.

Words to Understand

Nonprofit organizations are organizations that are not-for-profit and exist to benefit the public.

Abortions are the termination of a pregnancy, whether through natural or surgical means.

Nongovernmental organizations are organizations created to benefit their members or a certain population. They are usually not-for-profit and help to advance underprivileged groups.

Humanitarian aid is assistance provided to a population, usually in response to some sort of crisis.

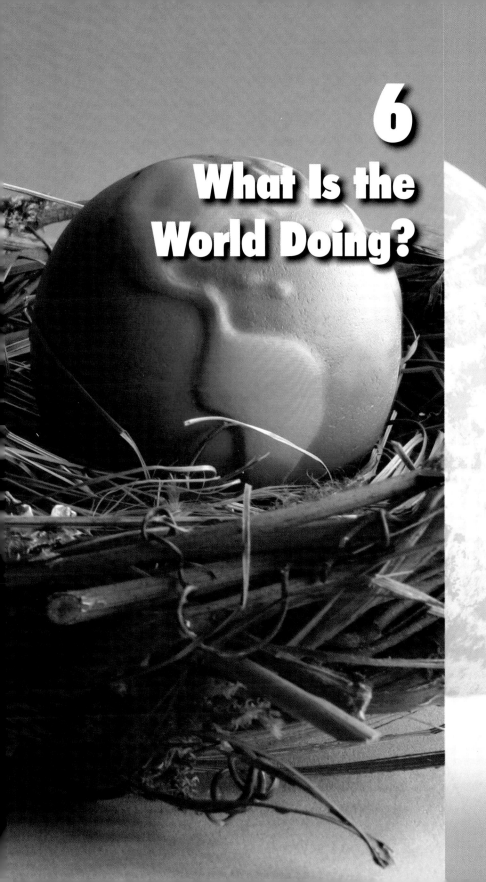

6

What Is the World Doing?

The world is by no means sitting back while more and more people squeeze onto the planet. **Nonprofit organizations**, governments and government agencies, and individuals are doing their part to fight the negative effects of population growth. Their actions take the form of education programs, data collection, fundraising, providing health care for those in need, or other things. People who are more removed from the effects of population growth and who have not yet faced large-scale food shortages or lack of health care are beginning to understand the problems an overpopulated Earth is dealing with. What's more, millions of people are acting to solve these problems, and are succeeding.

UN Initiatives

The United Nations is an international organization made up of almost 200 countries. In 1945, the founding countries of the UN pledged to work toward international security, economic development, human rights, and other global issues. One of its main purposes is to provide a place for countries in conflict to work out their differences peacefully, without turning to violence and war.

Today, in addition to all of these goals, the UN also deals with the issue of population growth. One part of the UN called the United Nations Fund for Population Activities (UNFPA) works to address issues surrounding population growth, specifically health and human rights concerns. Its mission statement reads,

> UNFPA, the United Nations Population Fund, is an international development agency that promotes the right of every woman, man and child to enjoy a life of health and equal opportunity. UNFPA supports countries in using population data for policies and programmes to reduce poverty and to ensure that every pregnancy is wanted, every birth is safe, every young person is free of HIV/AIDS, and every girl and woman is treated with dignity and respect.

The organization works around the world. They focus on 150 nations in four regions in particular—Latin America and the Caribbean; sub-Saharan Africa; the Arab States, Europe, and Central Asia; and Asia and the Pacific.

UNFPA plays a big role in gathering data on population for the UN. Every year, it puts together numbers on population trends such as growth, distribution, and density. As UNFPA realizes, accurate and up-to-date information on population helps both the UN and governments figure out how to help people affected by food or water shortages, HIV/AIDS, lack of health care, or a host of other problems brought on or made worse by population growth. Historical and current population data also allows for predictions of future population trends, and helps us figure out the best way to approach problems in the future.

UNFPA supports many types of programs. It focuses heavily on reproductive health and the education of

The United Nations, headquartered in New York City, has engineered a variety of programs and policies administered worldwide to address issues of human rights and environmental policies.

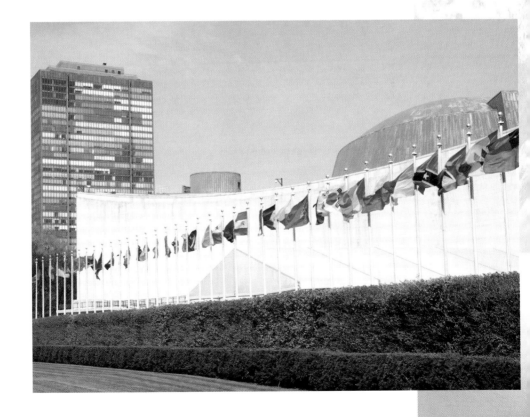

women and men on birth control and other forms of family planning. As a major international organization, it can help local and national governments make sure that addressing health problems related to population are part of their policymaking, so that millions of people world-wide can be helped by their own governments rather than by an outside organization. UNFPA fully supports what it calls a "culturally sensitive approach," which means that it respects the different cultural views and ideas that people have about population issues. It operates on the belief that the best and most effective way to tackle a problem such as reproductive health in Africa is to understand and work with the people who are being helped. No one wants to have an idea that they don't agree with forced on them, so UNFPA tries to find ways to work with communities rather than against them.

Every year, UNFPA releases a State of the World Population report, which details the year's population growth, its health effects, and the efforts made to reduce the consequences of an increasing population. It also publishes a youth supplement to the report, making its findings available to younger readers. Both reports provide an important resource for anyone looking for information on population, from individuals concerned about health crises to governments wishing to help their citizens.

Population Policies

The populations of different regions and countries are often very different from one another. In one area of the world, rapid urbanization might be the major problem, but in another, a shortage of food might be the most important issue. Demographics also vary across borders. Some nations have come up with official population policies so that they can more easily work toward a sustainable and healthy population.

The most famous policy on population is probably the one established in China. In 1979, the Chinese government decided to put a policy into place that limited the number of children each couple could have. Parents in more densely populated cities could have one child, while couples in rural areas could sometimes have up to two. The policy included laws that rewarded couples who followed it—money and better child care, among other things— and punishments for those who didn't. There have been reports of forced **abortions**, but China's official policy opposes them and focuses instead on rewards. Although it is highly controversial, it has generally been successful as far as reducing population growth and meeting China's

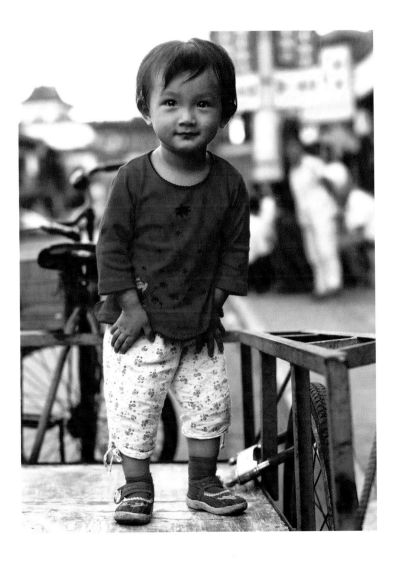

China is the world's most populated country. The Chinese government implemented controversial population policies in 1979 to limit the number of children per couple in order to curb population growth.

goal of stopping growth in the first half of the twenty-first century. China still has an enormous population, but it is growing more slowly, as women have fewer children than they did half a century ago.

Less-industrial developing countries also have population policies. In 2007, 66 percent of all countries in Africa had policies aimed at managing population growth. Kenya, for example, initiated one in the late 1960s that focuses on limiting population to the number of resources the country has in order to keep its population at a manageable level. It is different than China's policy, however, because it does not legally limit the size of families, and leaves it to individual choice. By increasing education about family planning and contraceptives, especially through local health offices, the average number of children each woman gives birth to has dropped by half since the 1980s. Although developing countries often run into problems implementing their policies, and have significant obstacles to face such as HIV/AIDS and poverty, places such as Kenya seem to be moving in the right direction.

Many countries in Africa are especially devastated by the HIV/AIDS epidemic, because they are hard-pressed to devote already scant resources to prevention and treatment programs. As a result, many international humanitarian aid organizations end up filling this gap. For example, organizations such as the UN, and WHO play a major role in providing funding and resources for HIV/AIDS prevention programs worldwide.

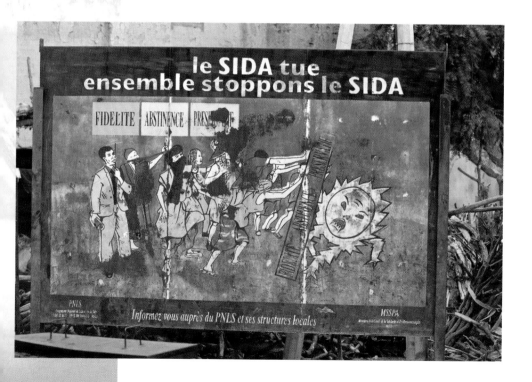

Official population policies in developed countries are more rare. Most policies were created in the last quarter of the twentieth century, when population was beginning to stabilize in developed countries. Government regulations limiting population were therefore less of a priority than in countries whose population increases showed no sign of slowing down. In 2007, the UN released a World Population Policy report that found that twenty-two countries, mostly in Europe, had policies meant to deal with falling populations. Since growth rate has slowed or even stopped, a shrinking population is a real possibility for some countries, which has the potential to be as problematic as growth. The main concern of these countries is for their economies: the number of people in the workforce will drop, with economic consequences. To keep their economies going, some nations have been increasing the legal retirement age or have created programs to push women to join the workforce.

Education

Education is an important part of combating the health and environmental impacts of population growth because not everyone is aware of this global problem. People's actions make a difference, whether they send money to feed a community across the globe or work at an NGO dealing with pollution. However, if people don't know about an issue, they certainly can't decide to do something about it. Education can also prevent potential health issues from becoming problems, or can reverse damage already done. Training people in how to grow crops sustainably will result in more food, or teaching them how to properly dispose of sewage will prevent water contamination.

When governments make an effort through policymaking to limit the growth of their countries' population, they often turn to education. Providing education for citizens on family planning methods and where to find contraception are important aspects of limiting fertility. Many countries have educational programs aimed at adolescents in order to prevent pregnancies in women under twenty. Eighty percent of the countries that provided information to the UN for its report had policies that were focused on adolescent pregnancy, providing information for schools, setting up counseling programs, and giving money to **nongovernmental organizations** (NGOs), among other things. Countries that turn to education have a high chance of success at limiting their population growth. In Tunisia, which had an extremely high level of fertility in the 1960s, the government launched a program to educate Tunisians on family planning, while providing them with access to it at the same time. Today, the country has reached the replacement level of fertility.

Governments aren't the only organizations educating people about the health issues related to population growth. Intergovernmental organizations such as the UN, the World Bank, and the WHO (part of the UN) all have divisions that provide education about the health consequences of pollution, inadequate food and water, and other issues having ties to population growth. Because they bring together many countries under one organization, they are good sources for knowledge that applies to global problems and solutions such as population growth and health.

Hundreds of other organizations that work internationally or dedicate themselves to a single country or region also work toward educating the public and policymakers on health and population growth. The Population Reference Bureau (PRB) is dedicated to issues surrounding population growth, including health. PRB, for example, is a resource for individuals interested in learning about population growth, policymakers, educators, journalists, and others through publications and a Web site. It also does on-the-ground education, setting up workshops to educate about the same topics. Heifer International, an American-based group that does work around the world, is another nonprofit organization that focuses on both action and education, helping people fight hunger and malnutrition brought on in part by overpopulation. Part of their mission includes educating Americans about the world's food problems, and teaching communities in the United States and other countries how to overcome health, economic, and social problems relating to food shortages.

Organizations independent of health care or population growth are also realizing the global importance of population trends. The International Institute for Applied Systems Analysis (IIASA) in Austria has a program dedicated to studying population data and the consequences of population change on the world. IIASA takes a scientific approach to understanding population, publishing articles and books and providing a place for experts to collect information and talk to one another.

Real People

Shi Guangzhi is a silkworm farmer, in Sichuan Province, China. Her first task of every day is checking on her silkworms.

The silkworms eat mulberry leaves in large wicker trays stacked in her kitchen. Guangzhi picks through them carefully and inspects them. She must check their progress toward adulthood carefully, because the cocoons they spin are very important to her.

In fact, these silkworms mean everything to Guangzhi. The fibers they spin have lifted her and hundreds of women like her out of poverty, with the help of Heifer International. Since Guangzhi began working with Heifer International just two years ago, she has quadrupled her family's annual income.

www.heifer.org

Obstacles

Population growth, and its resulting health consequences, is one of the biggest problems we face today. There is no escaping the effects of adding millions of people to the globe every day, although some people are certainly more sheltered from those effects than others. Unfortunately, the people with the best resources available to do something about the effects of population growth are often the ones least affected by it. Those who live in developed areas of the world often have more money and access to ways to spread information and supplies to the places that need them most. Yet these people are the ones most removed from the greatest dangers that population growth poses and are sometimes the most unaware, since they live in countries that may even be declining in population. Citizens of developing countries are by no means unable to help themselves or unwilling to do so, but they must deal with poverty, a lack of education, and enormous health problems that require more resources and effort than they can devote.

Governments and politics also can stand in the way of making more progress against the health effects of population growth. In many cases, the governments of countries with rapidly growing populations are more interested in other things. Some governments have the best interests of their countries in mind, and choose to pour money and workers into developing economies to boost the standard of life of the people who live there. In other cases, governments are corrupt, and officials want

THE WORLD BANK

The World Bank is an international organization that focuses on the economic and financial development of the world's least-developed countries. It offers loans and expertise to help nations develop in areas such as education, health, and business. One-hundred eighty-five countries are members of the World Bank, which is run by a President and Board of Directors. It has faced a lot of criticism since its creation in 1945, but has seen both failures and successes.

to make money and gain power rather than work for the public. In any case, population growth is a difficult crisis to alleviate. Governments must be efficient, well run, and have access to a source of funding if they truly want to improve the health of citizens. Governments in turmoil, or those dealing with other issues, have a hard time dealing with population growth whether or not they have the country's best interests in mind.

Other, more immediate crises also steal the spotlight from the problem of population growth. It is necessary and sometimes easier to address the emergencies that require pressing attention, such as the death and destruction caused by a massive hurricane or the HIV/AIDS epidemic, rather than solve the underlying population growth problem. **Humanitarian aid** to victims of visible crises gets more media attention, donated money, and a quick response from world leaders. It is easy to recognize that a city shaken by an earthquake needs help; it is slightly more difficult to understand that countries around the world need to stop their populations from growing, much less come up with a way to make that happen.

The problem of population growth is an enormous one, and requires dedication, time, money, and cooperation to solve. International organizations and nonprofit groups must work well with local governments and citizens to figure out how to appropriately provide education and help that will last long into the future. There is always the danger that an outsider helping someone who is malnourished or suffering from lead poisoning will not understand the solution, and come up with one that is wrong for the people whose health is affected by growth. In the end, there is no magic solution for everyone on Earth; we must work country-by-country and area-by-area to address the unique situation in each.

Ask the Doctor

Q: What can I do to help starving people?

There are many things you can do to help people who are suffering from a lack of necessities. The cheapest is probably to write to your government and ask them to increase aid to poor developing countries. The next step up after this is to give money or even your labor to the NGO aid organizations that have made it their work to help people. But remember, even if you live a rich country, there are still people who are hungry, even in your hometown. Don't forget to give your time and money to local aid organizations as well.

STRAIGHT FROM THE SOURCE

The IIASA is one organization that is doing research on global population growth. It is an important source of scientific data on population trends that has the potential to influence governmental policies and educational action.

Human population matters for sustainable development in two important ways. First, it is an agent of change, inducing many of the environmental, economic and social changes in the world that give rise to concerns about the sustainability of current development paths. Second, the human population and its living conditions are the ultimate objects of development, with long-term human survival, health and well-being serving as criteria for judging whether development is sustainable or not.

Since the early days of IIASA, its population research activities (POP) have dealt with both the determinants and the consequences of population trends on a global, regional, national and sub-national level.

Beyond its firm foundation in formal demography POP research has greatly benefited from the interdisciplinary setting at IIASA, which has been a constant stimulus to look beyond the boundaries of demography and respond to the questions of how alternative future population trends may influence the rest of the world and how in turn changes in society, economy and the natural environment feed back on the human population by influencing its health and mortality, its migratory patterns, and its reproductive behavior.

What Do You Think?

• What are some specific ways a decrease in the rate of population growth can lead to sustainability?

• Why is it important that organizations like this one are interdisciplinary and focus on many different aspects of population growth and environmental concerns at once?

Find Out More

To learn more about these topics, check out these Web sites:

Heifer International
www.heifer.org

UNFPA
www.unfpa.org

IIASA
www.iiasa.ac.at

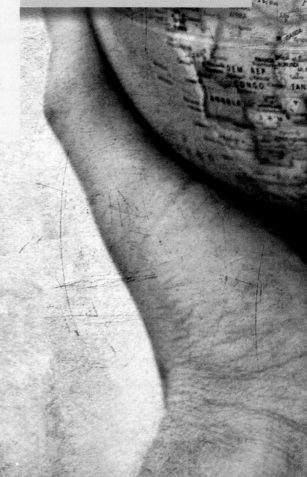

Here's what you need to know

- If you want to help, you can start by taking action in your own home or school.
- It's important to think on a global level, and to consider all of the consequences, positive and negative, of your action or inaction.
- You can also help by educating others, volunteering your time in a nonprofit organization, or giving money to an organization.

Words to Understand

A **global citizen** is a person who expands the definition of their citizenship beyond their home country, instead considering themselves a member of the global community.

Fundraising is the raising of money, usually in large quantities, that benefits a greater cause.

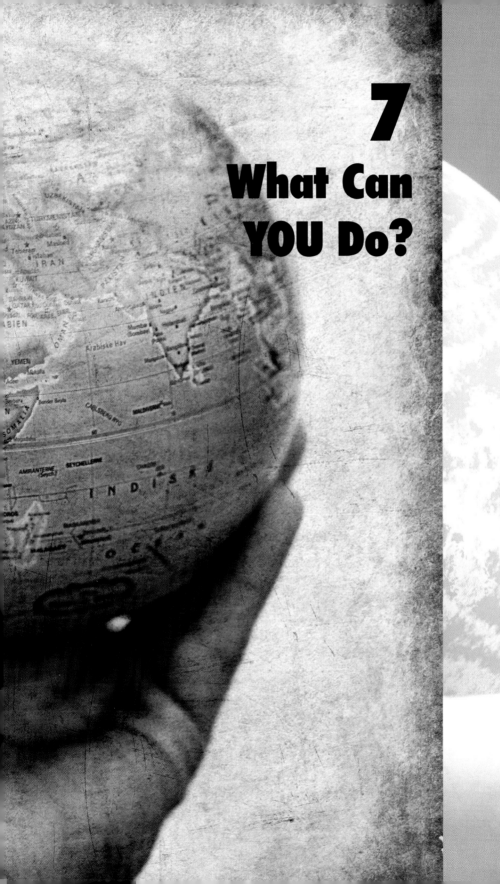

7

What Can YOU Do?

Because population growth is such a global issue, it can seem overwhelming. As an individual person, you might not think that anything you could do would help someone across the globe. But small changes in how you live do make a difference, especially if you convince others to make the same ones. You can even decide to act on a larger scale, and make a personal contribution to the fight against population growth. Simply learning about the issue is the first step toward effecting change.

Acting Locally

Population growth is a worldwide issue, which means it concerns all parts of the globe, even your own town or city. Just because you might not have experienced food shortages or difficulty obtaining medicine when you were sick doesn't mean that the rising number of people on the planet doesn't affect you, or won't in the future. You might start noticing the stress that increasing numbers of people puts on hospitals and doctors, stretching their resources thin between so many people. Or you might become aware of how much pollution large populations create through waste.

One place to start taking action is in your home or school. Start thinking about the effects that your actions have on the people surrounding you. Does your house use pesticides? If your entire neighborhood uses pesticides to

THE PEACE CORPS

The Peace Corps is an organization founded in 1961 that is dedicated to promoting peace in developing countries. It has sent thousands of Americans all over the planet to work with issues ranging from health, to environmental problems, to economic development. Volunteers travel to the field and get a real-life understanding of the problems they want to help solve, gaining skills and experience at the same time as helping others. So far, the Peace Corps has sent almost 200,000 volunteers to about 140 different countries.

treat lawns or parks, all of those chemicals run off into nearby streams, rivers, lakes, and oceans. The pollution created by so many people using pesticides leads to a buildup of harmful toxins in the water. In places where water is treated before being sent to houses and businesses, the likelihood that chemicals will contaminate drinking water is low. But if water is not treated before being consumed, the risk dramatically increases. There is also a real chance that fish that will eventually be consumed by people have also ingested some of the toxins from lawn pesticides, potentially spreading sickness.

Taking personally the effects of population growth on the Earth and all the people who inhabit it means that you probably have a good grasp of the problems we face. Carefully considering how many children you have someday is one of the first steps in being a responsible **global citizen**. Whether or not people have the right to tell others how many children to have is up for debate, but freely choosing to limit the number of children you have, or adopting one or more children, should be on everyone's mind in light of population growth. A stable population means a healthier one for those living on the Earth. When there are too many people, many of them suffer from the health consequences of malnutrition, pollution, water shortages, and lack of health care.

Global Awareness

Just learning about the issues surrounding population growth puts people in a better position to do something about it. Once you know that population growth is affecting the health of billions of people because of problems such as food shortages, unclean water, and pollution, you can learn how to do something about it. Educating others about what you already know spreads knowledge and might inspire someone else to act, too. This can be as simple as striking up a conversation with your friends about it, doing a school project about the health impacts

Did You Know?

Coal-burning power plants emit mercury into the air, where it stays until rain brings it down into water sources such as rivers, lakes, and oceans. Many fish accumulate mercury in their bodies, which is a health hazard to people around the world, especially those who depend on fish to survive.

of population growth, or starting a club to talk about the issues that concern you.

Donating money is also a good place to start. Every small amount that a person donates helps international organizations and nonprofits that are working in the field pay for medical care for AIDS victims, education about contraception, or cleaning up a polluted stream. Heifer International, for example, offers shares of livestock animals for as little as ten dollars. Your money goes directly to buying animals that will help families and communities in countries that face hunger such as Peru, Thailand, the United States, and Canada.

On an even larger scale, **fundraising** multiplies the amount of money one individual can donate. After choosing a charity, you can have fun and make a difference at the same time by hosting a fundraising event. It could be anything from a bake sale to a bottle drive, or something more creative. The bigger and more organized it is, the more money you'll collect and you'll feel like you're making a difference in people's lives. Successful fundraisers can earn hundreds or even thousands of dollars to send to an organization in need.

Besides thinking about how your actions affect your friends, family, and neighbors, considering how they impact people on the other side of the world is just as important. Think about what you eat, for example. Raising cows for beef uses up much more water, land, and grain than chickens, pigs, or vegetables. Limiting your consumption of the foods that use up the most resources helps to save some for the people who really need the water, land, and crops that livestock use.

Ask the Doctor

Q: Where is the best place to help?

There is no one good place to give your time and money to. There are many organizations out there all working toward many different worthy goals, and through many different means. The best option for you is to find one that personally appeals to you, with goals and methods that you personally approve of and support.

Action on All Levels

If you decide that population growth and its consequences, whether they involve health, the environment, or another concern, are issues that you really want to do something about actively, there are lots of options. Donating time and effort through volunteer work is definitely appreciated by groups that work with global health care, and will teach you even more about the issues you're passionate about. Many international organizations have local branches that you can volunteer at, either on a weekly basis or for a few months at a time.

It's possible to dedicate even more time to this issue, if you're really willing to tackle population growth. Volunteering for months or years at a time to work on service projects in the field is one option. Participating in programs such as the Peace Corps, which sends people to developing nations to work toward solving global issues such as health and population growth is a great opportunity to actively help the people hardest hit by growth. Setting a goal of working for a nonprofit group or an international organization that deals with population growth can be something to work toward in the future as well.

So whether you choose to donate money, educate others, or work in the field, there are lots of things you can decide to do to tackle population growth. The world needs answers now, before the problems get even worse. Fortunately, there is an end to population growth in sight, but slowing or stopping it depends on people's actions now. The health of literally billions of people depends on how many people are added to the planet every year, so we only stand to gain from fighting lack of health care, shortages of water, malnutrition and starvation, pollution, or population growth itself.

Did You Know?

Approximately 187,000 people have volunteered in the Peace Corps since it was founded in 1961.

STRAIGHT FROM THE SOURCE

The Peace Corps is one way to dedicate yourself to the health issues related to population growth. The organization offers many ways to help people around the world, health being one of them. Here's how it describes itself:

Peace Corps Volunteers work in health projects providing maternal and child health services, nutrition and hygiene messages, organizational support at community clinics, and education about prevention of infections and vaccine-preventable diseases. Volunteers also help expand access to clean water and improve sanitation by advising communities how to build and maintain wells and latrines. By focusing on prevention, human capacity building, and education, Peace Corps Volunteers help improve basic healthcare at the grassroots level, where their impact can be the most significant and where health needs are most pressing. In helping communities take more responsibility for their own healthcare, Volunteers work to ensure the sustainability of their projects.

In addition to working on basic health issues, Volunteers address the impact from the global pandemic of HIV/AIDS. Volunteers in HIV/AIDS education and prevention train youth as peer educators, collaborate with community leaders to develop appropriate education strategies, provide support to children orphaned by HIV/AIDS, and develop programs that provide support to families and communities affected by the disease. Volunteers do not provide direct medical care.

What Do You Think?

• Do you think it's important for members of developed countries to go volunteer abroad in programs like the Peace Corps? Why or why not?

• What are some things these volunteers can accomplish that local workers might not be able to? Why do you think this is?

Find Out More

To find out more about the Peace Corps, go to:

Peace Corps
www.peacecorps.gov

For More Information on Health & the Environment

Books

Gordon, Bruce, Richard Mackay and Eva Rehfuess. *Inheriting the World: The Atlas of Children's Health and the Environment.* World Health Organization, 2004.

Ho, Mun S. and Chris P. Nielsen, eds. *Clearing the Air: the Health and Economic Damages of Air Pollution in China.* Cambridge, MA: MIT Press, 2007.

Kusinitz, Marc. *Poisons and Toxins.* New York: Chelsea House Publications, 1992.

MacDonald, John J. *Environments for Health.* New York: Earthscan Publications, 2006.

McCally, Michael, ed. *Life Support: The Environment and Human Health.* Cambridge, MA: MIT Press, 2002.

Nadakavukaren, Anne. *Our Global Environment: a Health Perspective.* 6th edition. New York: Waveland Press, 2005.

Nakaya, Andrea C. *Is Air Pollution a Serious Threat to Health?* New York: Greenhaven Press, 2004.

Netzley, Patricia D. *Contemporary Issues: Issues in the Environment.* New York: Lucent Books, 1997.

Vesley, Donald. Human *Health and the Environment: A Turn of the Century Perspective.* New York: Springer, 1999.

Web Sites

Air Pollution
health.nih.gov/result.asp/19

Air Quality
www.epa.gov/airnow/

CDC: Environmental Health
www.cdc.gov/Environmental/

EPA: Environmental Kids Club
www.epa.gov/kids/

The Green Squad
www.nrdc.org/greensquad/intro/intro_1.asp

Health and Environmental Linkages Initiative
www.who.int/heli/en/

International Year of Sanitation
www.who.int/water_sanitation_health/hygiene/iys/
about/en/index3.html

Kids for Saving Earth
www.kidsforsavingearth.org/index_low.html

Library of Congress Environmental; Photographs
memory.loc.gov/ammem/award97/icuhtml/aephome.html

Public Health and the Environment
www.who.int/phe/en/

Teen Ink
www.teenink.com/Environment/index.php

Toxic Household Cleaners
www.tutorials.com/08/0858/0858.asp

United Nations Population Fund
www.unfpa.org/

Water and Sanitation Quiz
www.unicef.org/voy/explore/wes/1883_wes_quiz.php

Glossary of Environmental Health–Related Terms

When you're reading about environmental health, especially in some of the more technical government reports, you may encounter many unfamiliar medical terms. This glossary can help you better understand the words scientists and other experts use when talking about the effects of environmental pollution on human health.

Absorption
The process of taking in; for a person or an animal, this refers to a substance getting into the body through the eyes, skin, stomach, intestines, or lungs. Chemicals can be absorbed into the bloodstream after breathing or swallowing. Chemicals can also be absorbed through the skin, into the bloodstream, and then transported to other organs. Not all chemicals breathed, swallowed, or touched are absorbed.

Acute
Occurring over a short time, usually a few minutes or hours. An acute exposure only lasts for up to 14 days; it can result in short-term or long-term health effects. An acute effect happens a short time after exposure.

Additive Effect
The body's response to exposure to multiple substances that equals the sum of responses of all the individual substances added together.

Adverse Health Effect
A change in body function or cell structure that might lead to disease or health problems.

Ambient
Surrounding. Ambient air usually means outdoor air (as opposed to indoor air).

Analyte

A chemical for which a sample (such as water, air, blood, urine, or another substance) is tested and measured in the laboratory. For example, if the analyte is mercury, the laboratory test will determine the amount of mercury in the sample.

Antagonistic Effect

A biologic response to exposure to multiple substances that is less than would be expected if the known effects of the individual substances were added together.

Aquatic Ecosystem

A community of organisms that live together in a body of water and are interdependent.

Aquifer

A geological formation where the spaces between rock particles, sand, or gravel are completely filled with water. Water pumped from aquifers is referred to as "groundwater".

Background Level

A typical or average level of a chemical in the environment. Background often refers to naturally occurring or uncontaminated levels. Background levels in one region of the world may be different than those in other areas.

Bedrock

The solid rock underneath surface soils.

Biodegradation

Decomposition or breakdown of a substance through the action of microorganisms (such as bacteria or fungi) or other natural, physical processes (such as sunlight).

Biologic Indicators of Exposure Study

A study that uses medical tests and other markers of exposure in human body fluids or tissues to confirm human exposure to a hazardous substance.

Biological Monitoring

Measuring chemicals, hormone levels, or other substances in biological materials (blood, urine, breath, or hair) as a measure of chemical exposure and health in humans or animals. A blood test for lead is an example of biological monitoring.

Biologic Uptake

The transfer of substances from the environment to plants, animals, and humans.

Biomedical Testing

Testing of persons to find out whether a change in a body function might have occurred because of exposure to a hazardous substance in the environment.

Biota

Plants and animals in an environment. Some of these plants and animals might be sources of food, clothing, or medicines for people.

Body Burden

The total amount of a chemical in the body. Some chemicals build up in the body because they are stored in body organs like fat or bone or are eliminated very slowly.

Cancer

Any one of a group of diseases that occur when cells in the body become abnormal and grow or multiply out of control.

Cancer Risk

The theoretical risk for getting cancer if exposed to a substance every day for 70 years (a lifetime exposure). The true risk might be lower.

Carcinogen

A substance that causes cancer.

Case Study
A medical evaluation of one person or a small group of people to gather information about specific health conditions and past exposures.

Case-Control Study
A study in which a group of people with a disease (cases) are compared to people without the disease (controls) to see if their past exposures to chemicals or other risk factors were different.

Central Nervous System (CNS)
The part of the nervous system that includes the brain and the spinal cord.

Chronic
Occurring over a long period of time, several weeks, months, or years.

Chronic Exposure
Contact with a substance that occurs over a long time (more than a year).

Cluster Investigation
A review of an unusual number, real or perceived, of health events (for example, reports of cancer) grouped together in time and location. Cluster investigations are designed to confirm case reports; determine whether they represent an unusual disease occurrence; and, if possible, explore possible causes and contributing environmental factors.

Cohort Study
A study in which a group of people with a past exposure to chemicals or other risk factors are followed over time and their disease experience compared to that of a group of people without the exposure.

Comparison Value (CV)

Calculated concentration of a substance in air, water, food, or soil that is unlikely to cause harmful (adverse) health effects in exposed people. The CV is used as a screening level during the public health assessment process. Substances found in amounts greater than their CVs might be selected for further evaluation in the public health assessment process.

Composite Sample

A sample which is made by combining samples from two or more locations. The sample can be of water, soil, or another substance found in the environment.

Concentration

The amount of one substance dissolved or contained in a given amount of another substance. For example, sea water has a higher concentration of salt than fresh water does.

Contaminant

Any substance found somewhere (for example, the environment, the human body, or food) where it is not normally found. Contaminants are usually referred to in a negative sense and include substances that spoil food, pollute the environment, or cause other adverse effects.

Delayed Health Effect

A disease or an injury that happens as a result of exposure that might have occurred in the past.

Dermal

Having to do with the skin. For example, dermal absorption means absorption through the skin.

Dermal Contact

Touching the skin.

Detection Limit

The smallest amount of substance that a laboratory test can reliably measure in a sample of air, water, soil, or other medium.

Dose

The amount of substance to which a person is exposed. Dose is a measurement of exposure and is often expressed as milligram (amount) per kilogram (a measure of body weight) per day (a measure of time) when people eat or drink contaminated water, food, or soil. In general, the greater the dose, the greater the likelihood of an effect. An "exposure dose" is how much of a substance is encountered in the environment. An "absorbed dose" is the amount of a substance that actually got into the body through the eyes, skin, stomach, intestines, or lungs. For radioactive chemicals, dose is the amount of energy from radiation that is actually absorbed by the body. This is not the same as the measurement of the amount of radiation in the environment.

Dose-Response Relationship

The relationship between the amount of exposure to a substance and the resulting changes in body function or health.

Environmental Media and Transport Mechanism

Environmental media include water, air, soil, plants, and animals. Transport mechanisms move contaminants from the source to points where human exposure can occur. The environmental media and transport mechanism is the second part of an exposure pathway.

EPA

United States Environmental Protection Agency.

Epidemiology

The study of the occurrence and causes of health effects in human populations. An epidemiological study often

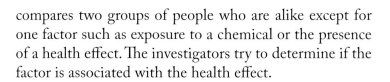

compares two groups of people who are alike except for one factor such as exposure to a chemical or the presence of a health effect. The investigators try to determine if the factor is associated with the health effect.

Exposure
Contact with a chemical by swallowing, breathing, or direct contact (such as through the skin or eyes). Exposure may be either short term (acute) or long term (chronic).

Exposure Assessment
The process of finding out how people come into contact with a hazardous substance, how often and for how long they were in contact with the substance, and how much of the substance they were in contact with.

Exposure-Dose Reconstruction
A method of estimating the amount of people's past exposure to hazardous substances. Computer and approximation methods are used when past information is limited, not available, or missing.

Exposure Investigation
The collection and analysis of information from an environmental site and biologic tests to determine whether people have been exposed to hazardous substances.

Exposure Pathway
The route a substance takes from its source (where it began) to its end point (where it ends), and how people can come into contact with (or get exposed to) it along the way. An exposure pathway has five parts: a source of contamination (such as an abandoned business); an environmental media and transport mechanism (such as movement through groundwater); a point of exposure (such as a private well); a route of exposure (eating, drinking, breathing, or touching), and a receptor population (people potentially or actually exposed). When all five parts are present, the exposure pathway is termed a completed exposure pathway.

Exposure Registry

A system of the ongoing follow-up of people who have had documented environmental exposures.

Feasibility Study (FS)

A study that compares different ways to clean up a contaminated site. The feasibility study recommends one or more actions to remediate the site.

Geographic Information System (GIS)

A mapping system that uses computers to collect, store, manipulate, analyze, and display data. For example, GIS can show the concentration of a contaminant within a community in relation to points of reference such as streets and homes.

Gradient

The change in a property over a certain distance. For example, lead can accumulate in surface soil near a road due to automobile exhaust. As you move away from the road, the amount of lead in the surface soil decreases. This change in the lead concentration with distance from the road is called a gradient.

Groundwater

Water beneath the earth's surface in aquifers (as opposed to surface water)

Half-Life

The time it takes for half the original amount of a substance to disappear. In the environment, the half-life is the time it takes for half the original amount of a substance to disappear when it is changed to another chemical by bacteria, fungi, sunlight, or other chemical processes. In the human body, the half-life is the time it takes for half the original amount of the substance to disappear, either by being changed to another substance or by leaving the body. In the case of radioactive material, the half-life is the amount of time necessary for one-half the initial number of radioactive atoms to change or transform into another atom (that is normally not radioactive). After two-half lives, 25% of the original number of radioactive atoms remain.

Hazard
A source of potential harm from past, current, or future exposures.

Hazardous Waste
Potentially harmful substances that have been released or discarded into the environment.

Health Assessment for Contaminated Sites
Determination of actual or possible health effects due to environmental contamination or exposure. It includes a health-based interpretation of all the information known about the situation. The information may come from site investigations (environmental sampling and studies), exposure assessments, risk assessments, biological monitoring, or health effects studies. The health assessment is used to advise people on how to prevent or reduce their exposures, to determine what action to take to improve the situation, or the need for additional studies.

Health Effects Studies (related to contaminants)
Studies of the health of people who may have been exposed to contaminants. They include, but are not limited to, epidemiological studies, reviews of the health status of people in exposure or disease registries, and doing medical tests.

Health Registry
A record of people exposed to a specific substance (such as a heavy metal), or having a specific health condition (such as cancer or a communicable disease).

Incidence
The number of new cases of disease in a defined population over a specific time period.

Ingestion
Swallowing (such as through eating or drinking). After ingestion, chemicals may be absorbed into the blood and distributed throughout the body.

Inhalation
Breathing. People can take in chemicals by breathing contaminated air.

Interim Remedial Measure (IRM)
An action taken at a contaminated site to reduce the chances of human or environmental exposure to site contaminants. Interim remedial measures are planned and carried out before comprehensive remedial studies. They can prevent additional damage during the study phase, but don't interfere in any way with the need to develop a complete remedial program. An example of an interim remedial measure is removing drums of chemicals to a storage facility from a site that has drums sitting in an empty field.

In Vitro
In an artificial environment outside a living organism or body. For example, some tests are done on cell cultures or slices of tissue grown in the laboratory, rather than on a living animal.

In Vivo
Within a living organism or body. For example, when scientific research is done on whole animals, such as rats or mice.

Latency period
The period of time between exposure to something that causes a disease and the onset of the health effect. Cancer caused by chemical exposure may have a latency period of 5 to 40 years.

Leaching

As water moves through soils or landfills, chemicals in the soil may dissolve in the water, thereby contaminating the groundwater. This is called leaching.

Maximum Contaminant Level (MCL)

The highest (maximum) level of a contaminant allowed to go uncorrected by a public water system under federal or state regulations. Depending on the contaminant, allowable levels might be calculated as an average over time or might be based on individual test results. Corrective steps are implemented if the MCL is exceeded.

Media

Elements of a surrounding environment that can be sampled for contamination: usually soil, water, or air. Plants as well as humans (when sampling body substances such as blood or urine) and animals (such as sampling fish to update fish consumption advisories) can also be considered media. The singular of "media" is "medium."

Metabolism

All the chemical reactions that enable the body to work. For example, food is metabolized (chemically changed) to supply the body with energy. Chemicals can be metabolized by the body and made either more or less harmful.

Metabolite

Any product of metabolism.

Morbidity

Illness or disease. A morbidity rate for a certain illness is the number of people with that illness divided by the number of people in the population from which the illnesses were counted.

Mortality

Death. Usually the cause (a specific disease, a condition, or an injury) is stated along with this term.

Mutagen
A substance that causes mutations (genetic damage).

Mutation
A change (damage) to the DNA, genes, or chromosomes of living organisms.

Odor Threshold
The lowest concentration of a chemical that can be smelled. Different chemicals have different odor thresholds. Also, some people can smell a chemical at lower concentrations than others can.

Organic
Generally considered as originating from plants or animals, and made primarily of carbon and hydrogen. Scientists use the term organic to mean those chemical compounds which are based on carbon.

Permeability
The property of permitting liquids or gases to pass through. A highly permeable soil, such as sand, allows a liquid to pass through quickly. Clay has a low permeability.

Persistence
The quality of remaining for a long period of time (such as in the environment or the body). Persistent chemicals (such as DDT and PCBs) are not easily broken down.

Plume
An area of chemicals moving away from its source in a long band or column. A plume, for example, can be a column of smoke from a chimney or chemicals moving with groundwater.

Point of Exposure
The place where someone can come into contact with a substance present in the environment (see **Exposure Pathway**).

Population
A group or number of people living within a specified area or sharing similar characteristics (such as occupation or age).

Prevalence
The number of existing disease cases in a defined population during a specific time period.

Prevention
Actions that reduce exposure or other risks, keep people from getting sick, or keep disease from getting worse.

Protocol
The detailed plan for conducting a scientific procedure. A protocol for measuring a chemical in soil, water, or air describes the way in which samples should be collected and analyzed.

Radioisotope
An unstable or radioactive isotope of an element that can change into another element by giving off radiation.

Radionuclide
Any radioactive isotope of any element.

Receptor population
People who could come into contact with hazardous substance.

Registry
A systematic collection of information on persons exposed to a specific substance or having specific diseases.

Remedial Investigation (RI)
An in-depth study (including sampling of air, soil, water, and waste) of a contaminated site needing remediation to determine the nature and extent of contamination. The remedial investigation (RI) is usually combined with a feasibility study (FS).

Remediation

Correction or improvement of a problem, such as work that is done to clean up or stop the release of chemicals from a contaminated site. After investigation of a site, remedial work may include removing soil and/or drums, capping the site, or collecting and treating the contaminated fluids.

Risk

Risk is the possibility of injury, disease, or death. For example, for a person who has measles, the risk of death is one in one million.

Risk Assessment

A process which estimates the likelihood that exposed people may have health effects. The four steps of a risk assessment are: hazard identification (Can this substance damage health?); dose-response assessment (What dose causes what effect?); exposure assessment (How and how much do people come into contact with it?); and risk characterization (combining the other three steps to characterize risk and describe the limitations and uncertainties).

Risk Management (or Reduction)

The process of deciding how and to what extent to reduce or eliminate risk factors by considering the risk assessment, engineering factors (Can procedures or equipment do the job? For how long and how well?), social, economic, and political concerns.

Route of Exposure

The way in which a person may contact a chemical substance. For example, drinking (ingestion) and bathing (skin contact) are two different routes of exposure to contaminants that may be found in water. See **Exposure**.

Safe

Free from harm or risk. Exposure to a chemical usually has some risk associated with it, although the risk may be very small. However, many people use the word safe to mean something that has a very low risk or one that is acceptable to them.

Sample
A portion or piece of a whole. A selected subset of a population or subset of whatever is being studied. For example, in a study of people the sample is a number of people chosen from a larger population. (See **Population**.) An environmental sample (for example, a small amount of soil or water) might be collected to measure contamination in the environment at a specific location.

Sample Size
The number of units chosen from a population or an environment.

Solubility
The largest amount of a substance that can be dissolved in a given amount of a liquid, usually water. For a highly water-soluble compound, such as table salt, a lot can dissolve in water. Motor oil is only slightly soluble in water.

Solvent
A liquid capable of dissolving or dispersing another substance (for example, acetone or mineral spirits).

Source of Contamination
The place where a hazardous substance comes from, such as a landfill, waste pond, incinerator, storage tank, or drum. A source of contamination is the first part of an **Exposure Pathway**.

Special Populations
People who might be more sensitive or susceptible to exposure to hazardous substances because of factors such as age, occupation, sex, or behaviors (for example, cigarette smoking). Children, pregnant women, and older people are often considered special populations.

Stakeholder
A person, group, or community who has an interest in activities at a hazardous waste site.

Statistics
A branch of mathematics that deals with collecting, reviewing, summarizing, and interpreting data or information. Statistics are used to determine whether differences between study groups are meaningful.

Superfund
The United States' federal and state program that investigates and cleans up inactive, hazardous waste sites.

Surface Water
Water on the surface of the earth, such as in lakes, rivers, streams, ponds, and springs.

Synergistic effect
A biologic response to multiple substances where one substance worsens the effect of another substance. The combined effect of the substances acting together is greater than the sum of the effects of the substances acting by themselves.

Target Organ
An organ (such as the liver or kidney) that is specifically affected by a toxic chemical.

Teratogen
A substance that causes defects in development between conception and birth.

Toxic Agent
Chemical or physical (for example, radiation, heat, cold, microwaves) agents that, under certain circumstances of exposure, can cause harmful effects to living organisms.

Toxicology
The study of the harmful effects of substances on humans or animals.

Tumor
An abnormal mass of tissue that results from excessive cell division that is uncontrolled and progressive. Tumors perform no useful body function. Tumors can be either benign (not cancer) or malignant (cancer).

Volatile
Evaporating readily at normal temperatures and pressures. The air concentration of a highly volatile chemical can increase quickly in a closed room.

Volatile Organic Compound (VOC)
An organic chemical that evaporates readily. Petroleum products such as kerosene, gasoline, and mineral spirits contain VOCs. Chlorinated solvents, such as those used by dry cleaners or contained in paint strippers, are also VOCs.

Bibliography

Advameg. "Pollution Issues: Thermal Pollution". 2008. 20 June 2008. www.pollutionissues.com/Te-Un/Thermal-Pollution.html.

Buske, Lynda. "Number of Health Care Workers Lags Behind Population Growth." *Canadian Medical Association Journal*. 163.3 (2000): 323. 27 May 2008. www.pubmedcentral.nih.gov/articlerender.fcgi?artid=80325.

Food and Agriculture Organization of the United Nations. *FAO Focus: Women and Food Security*. 20 June 2008. www.fao.org/focus/e/women/green-e/htm.

Global Alliance for Improved Nutrition. "Malnutrition."
5 June 2008. www.gainhealth.org/press-centre/nutrition_
facts.

Harrison, Paul, Fred Pearce, and Peter Raven. "AAAS
Atlas of Population and Environment." American Association for the Advancement of Science, 2001. 25 May
2008. http://atlas.aaas.org/.

NOVA. "World in the Balance." PBS, 2004. www.pbs.
org/wgbh/nova/worldbalance/.

The Population Council. 8 June 2008. www.popcouncil.
org/index.html.

Population Reference Bureau. 2008. www.prb.org/.

Shapely, Dan. "U.S. Suburban Sprawl, by the Numbers."
The Daily Green, 27 March 2008. www.thedailygreen.
com/environmental-news/blogs/shapley/suburban-
sprawl-47032706.

United Nations. Department of Economic and Social
Affairs Population Division. 24 May 2008. www.un.org/
esa/population/unpop.htm.

U.S. Census Bureau. International Data Base. 23 May
2008. www.census.gov/ipc/www/idb/index.html.

U.S. Department of State. Bureau of East Asian and
Pacific Affairs. 8 June 2008. www.state.gov/r/pa/ei/
bgn/18902.htm.

"Why Water Matters." *World Ark Magazine.* May/June
2008: 10-17.

The World Bank. Disease Control Priorities Project. 2006.
27 May 2008. www.dcp2.org/pubs/GBD.

The World Bank. *Health, Nutrition, & Population.* 30 May 2008. go.worldbank.org/RQU0H5VGJ0.

World Overpopulation Awareness/ 24 May 2008. www.population-awareness.net/.

World Health Organization. *Water Sanitation and Health.* 1 June 2008. www.who.int/water_sanitation_health/en/.

World Water Council. 1 June 1008. www.worldwater-council.org/index.php?id=1&L=0.

Index

Picture Credits

Dreamstime.com
    Achilles: p. 45
    Bernardo69: p. 74
    Buttershug: p. 69
    Capturednuance p.25
    Corsec67: p. 62
    Costa007: p. 37
    Dreamshot63: p. 57
    Dsabo: p. 26
    Imantsu: p. 59
    Indiansummer: p. 23
    Janakadharmasena: p. 9
    Jckca: p. 15

Jeffbanke: p. 35
Kurhan: p. 29
Kydroon: p. 38
Mrincredible: p. 11
Pontuse: p. 17
Snehitdesign: p. 19
Thefinalmiracle: p. 47
Typhoonski: p. 71
Wysiwygfoto: p. 33
Yuri_arcurs: p. 83

Jupiterimages
pp. 12, 73